Lloyd Laver
1988

24-50

Surgical Diagnostic and Therapeutic Instruments

To Sue and Nicola,
for their unfailing patience
and support

Surgical Diagnostic and Therapeutic Instruments

JAN J. STANEK
MA, BM, FRCS
Private Practitioner, London

Blackwell Scientific Publications
OXFORD LONDON EDINBURGH
BOSTON PALO ALTO MELBOURNE

© 1986 by
Blackwell Scientific Publications
Editorial offices:
Osney Mead, Oxford OX2 0EL
8 John Street, London WC1N 2ES
23 Ainslie Place, Edinburgh EH3 6AJ
52 Beacon Street, Boston
　Massachusetts 02108, USA
667 Lytton Avenue, Palo Alto
　California 94301, USA
107 Barry Street, Carlton
　Victoria 3053, Australia

All rights reserved. No part of this
publication may be reproduced, stored
in a retrieval system, or transmitted,
in any form or by any means,
electronic, mechanical, photocopying,
recording or otherwise
without the prior permission of
the copyright owner

First published 1986

Set by Setrite Typesetters, Hong Kong
and printed and bound in Great Britain
at the University Press, Cambridge

DISTRIBUTORS

USA
Year Book Medical Publishers
35 East Wacker Drive
Chicago, Illinois 60601

Canada
Blackwell Mosby Book Distributors
120 Melford Drive, Scarborough
Ontario M1B 2X4

Australia
Blackwell Scientific Publications
(Australia) Pty Ltd
107 Barry Street
Carlton, Victoria 3053

British Library
Cataloguing in Publication Data

Stanek, Jan J.
　Surgical diagnostic and therapeutic
instruments.
　1. Medical instruments and apparatus
　I. Title
　610′.28　R856

ISBN 0-632-01177-7

Contents

Preface, vi

Introduction, vii

Acknowledgments, viii

Part 1 Diagnostic Instruments

1 Optical Instruments, 3
2 Ultrasound, Image Intensifier, CT Scan, Urodynamics, 21
3 Biopsies, 27

Part 2 Therapeutic Instruments

4 Vascular Access, 37
5 Drains and Splints, 49
6 Diathermy, Cryosurgery, Ultrasound, Dornier Lithotripter, 63
7 Sterilisation, Sutures, Gloves, Implants, 71

Part 3 Operative Instruments

8 General and Abdominal Surgery, 83
9 Gastrointestinal Stapling Instruments, 103
10 Plastic Surgery, 109
11 Urology, 117
12 Orthopaedics, 133
13 Vascular and Thoracic Surgery, 141
14 Neurosurgery, 153

General Reading, 159

Index, 161

Preface

Some years ago, as a Final Fellowship candidate, I became acutely aware of the need for a concise book on surgical instruments. I did not have one and have not found one since. During the next few years I formed the idea of writing such a book and eventually, with the support of the publishers, I committed myself to doing so.

I realise that my task is a daunting one, since I attempt to embrace a vast subject which is continually expanding. Operating instruments are no longer the only tools a surgeon has to master and I have included what I call therapeutic and diagnostic instruments in this book. These have become at least as important as the standard surgical instruments and are continually being improved and new ones introduced.

This book is intended not only for the young surgeon preparing for his or her Final surgical examination but also for those who are in everyday contact with these instruments: theatre nurses, senior surgeons, radiologists, physicians, anaesthetists and medical students. The scope of this book is limited and does not attempt to be authoritative; it outlines the basic principles only. I hope this book will bring some understanding of the subject and that it will give inspiration for new and better surgical tools which will ultimately benefit our patients.

JJS, London 1986

Introduction

No surgeon can fulfill himself in his profession without surgical instruments. The scalpel still remains one of his most important tools and is likely to stay for many years to come. However, the expansion of modern technology and enterprise has provided us with alternatives even to this most basic instrument. Diathermy, cryoprobe, ultrasound and even laser can replace the scalpel.

The application of modern synthetics has perfected suture materials, and catgut may soon become a thing of the past. Human organs are being replaced with artificial. Diagnostic tools have become as important to the surgeon as his surgical instruments. Accurate diagnosis is essential to an appropriate and effective treatment. Without the advent of fibrelight instruments we would not be able to visualise directly the duodenum, bile ducts, colon or even joints. Ultrasound and CT scan have provided us with a safe non-invasive tool of adequate accuracy which has changed the face of neurosurgery and obstetrics and is beginning to make impact on other specialities. Almost any hollow viscus or body cavity can be directly visualised, sampled or decompressed with the use of simple or complex apparatus. Thus major blood vessels or heart can be intubated for sampling, monitoring or transfusion. By the same route, arteries can be blocked, unblocked or even stretched.

The scope of modern surgical therapeutics is vast. For that reason it is no longer the domain of surgeons. Radiologists, anaesthetists, physicians and other specialists have learned to use, improve and expand this vast arsenal of tools. Many of them have become masters in their use and specialise in these procedures. To bring all this information into one book is a difficult task for one person and yet there is a need for such a book. Having reached a compromise I have written a book which deals with the very basic modern surgical diagnostic and therapeutic tools. The classification is mine and serves to preserve some order. As far as is possible each tool is shown in the form of a photograph, drawing or diagram. In some cases an historical note accompanies description, technique and indication of use. At the end of each section a list of general and specific references is given for those who wish to read further about the subject.

Acknowledgments

I am grateful to many individuals and companies who have made the publication of this book possible. The many excellent illustrations were generously supplied by Mr G.T.H. Mould of Downs Surgical plc, Mr Owen Meredith of AutoSuture UK Ltd., Mr Alan S. Costello of Vygon (UK) Ltd., Mr R.G. Urie of Franklin Medical, Mr Nigel Watkin of Codman Ltd, Mr Roger Gray of Key Med Ltd, Rimmer Brothers Ltd. and Karl Storz GmbH & Co.

Some of the instruments depicted are no longer manufactured and the reader is referred to up-to-date catalogues to ensure their availability.

I am also grateful for financial help towards research costs by Mr R.G. Urie of Franklin Medical and Mr Nigel Watkin of Codman Ltd.

The final drafts were typed by Miss Gill Baker and Miss Kathryn Nicholson, to whom I am grateful.

Some of the excellent drawings were made by Miss Ann Jeffries of Westminster Hospital Department of Medical Illustrations.

Finally, many thanks to Mr Peter Saugman of Blackwell Scientific Publications who made this book possible and to Mr Simon Rallison with his staff, who worked so hard to produce it.

Part 1　Diagnostic Instruments

Chapter 1　Optical Instruments

1.1　Laryngoscope and pharyngoscope
1.2　Bronchoscope
1.3　Mediastinoscope
1.4　Gastrointestinal endoscopy
　　　Oesophagoscope
　　　Gastroduodenoscope
　　　Proctoscope
　　　Sigmoidoscope
　　　Colonoscope
1.5　Choledoschoscope
1.6　Laparoscope
1.7　Arthroscope
1.8　Urological endoscopy
　　　Cysto-urethroscope
　　　Ureteroscope
　　　Nephroscope

1.1 Laryngoscope and pharyngoscope

The laryngoscope is an instrument designed to allow direct examination of the larynx and is most commonly used by anaesthetists for intubation. The most popular is the Macintosh pattern with a curved blade. This consists of a battery-containing handle with a curved blade attached to it by a hinge. A small electric bulb is situated halfway along the convex surface of the blade. The bulb is lit by moving the blade away from the handle to an approximately 90° angle, activating a switch. The blade is secured in this position by means of a spring-loaded lock. The blade is Z-shaped in cross-section to allow the tongue to be pushed to the opposite side of the mouth.

The Magill pattern laryngoscope has a straight and rather larger blade, which is designed to pass over the epiglottis. The Macintosh laryngoscope is held in the left hand and introduced to the right of the midline. The Z-shaped blade displaces the tongue to the left. The tip of the blade is advanced along the surface of the tongue towards the midline until the epiglottis comes into view and the vallecula is entered. The blade is then thrust upwards and away from the operator, lifting the tongue and epiglottis away from the posterior pharyngeal wall. This manoeuvre brings the larynx and vocal cords into view.

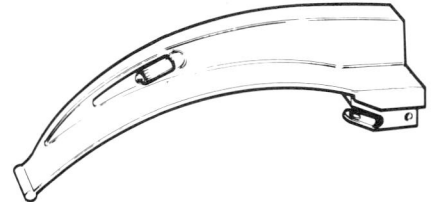

Fig.1 Macintosh laryngoscope blade (Downs)

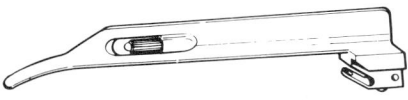

Fig.3 Magill laryngoscope blade (Downs)

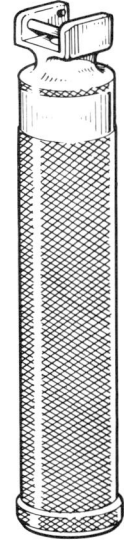

Fig.2 Anaesthetic laryngoscope handle (Downs)

4 DIAGNOSTIC INSTRUMENTS

The Negus pattern laryngoscope or oesophageal speculum is a diagnostic and therapeutic instrument, and resembles a short rigid bronchoscope or oesophagoscope with a handle. It is a short instrument with a rigid right-angled handle to allow the instrument to be thrust anteriorly and away from the operator during its insertion. A fibrelight illuminates the distal portion of the tube.

Jones, D.F. (1979) Endotracheal intubation. *Update*, Dec 1979, 1107-1117.
Dunkin, L.J. (1980) How to intubate. *British Journal of Hospital Medicine*, Jan 1980, 77-80.

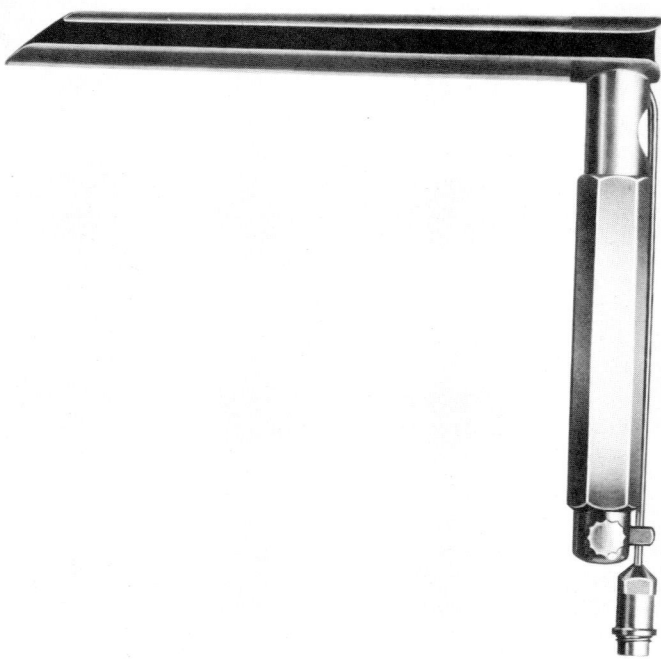

Fig.5 Operating pharyngoscope (Storz)

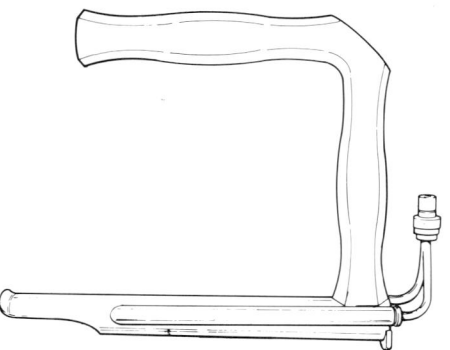

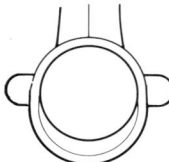

Fig.4 Negus laryngoscope and end of Negus laryngoscope (Downs)

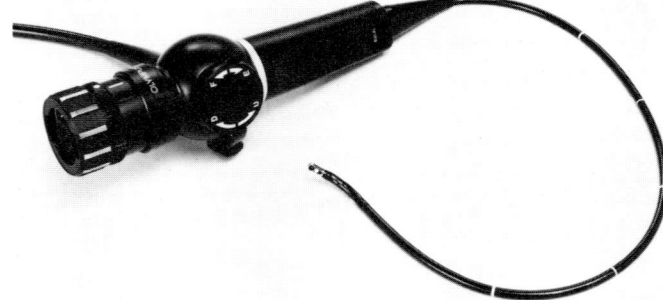

Fig.6 Olympus NPF-S4 side viewing flexible naso-pharyngoscope (Key Med)

1.2 Bronchoscope

The bronchoscope is a diagnostic as well as therapeutic instrument which allows direct visualisation of the trachea and the bronchial tree.

Prior to the introduction of the flexible fibreoptic bronchoscope, the use of a rigid bronchoscope was the domaine of thoracic and ENT surgeons. Today the majority of bronchoscopies are carried out by physicians interested in respiratory disease. However, the rigid bronchoscope is here to stay as it has some advantages over its flexible partner.

The rigid bronchoscope, such as the Negus or Chevalier–Jackson pattern, is a hollow tube, 40–45 cm long. There are several features which help to distinguish the rigid bronchoscope from the oesophagoscope. A bronchoscope usually has a rimmed bevelled end and the tube is conical (the diameter decreases towards the tip). It also has two slits on each side proximal to the tip to allow for the ventilation of upper bronchi which would otherwise be obstructed during examination. Some kind of air inlet is always provided and in the modern bronchoscope this takes the form of a venturi jet.

In cross section the adult bronchoscope is oval and its external diameter is about 11 mm at the tip.

Modern rigid bronchoscopes have a fibreoptic light source.

Before the introduction by Sanders in 1967 of the oxygen venturi

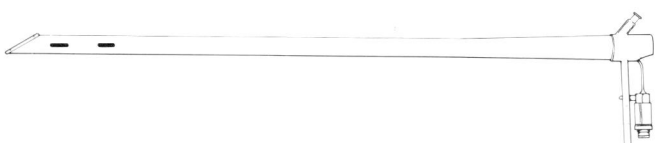

Fig. 7 Negus bronchoscope (Downs)

technique for ventilation, adequate ventilation during bronchoscopy was difficult and was achieved by supplying an intermittent air–oxygen mixture through a side tube at the proximal end of the bronchoscope. This always required closure of the proximal end of the instrument, necessitating a temporary interruption of the examination.

The venturi jet supplies oxygen through a small nozzle on the side of the instrument, with inflow controlled by an on/off valve.

The expanded oxygen draws in air through the main inlet and the lungs are thus inflated by air–oxygen mixture. Thus a gas flow of 6 l. min^{-1} can easily be achieved.

For routine bronchoscopy the patient lies supine, with a head rest. The neck is extended so that the chin points vertically upwards.

The three lateral fingers of the left hand are inserted into the mouth and hold the upper jaw, while the thumb and index fingers are used to support the instrument.

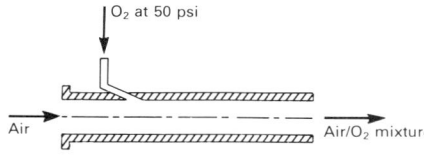

Fig. 8 Venturi jet

The bronchoscope is held in the right hand and, holding it almost vertically, its tip is inserted into the mouth to the right of the midline.

While the instrument is being inserted further, it is gradually brought downwards towards the operator as it follows the line of the tongue.

When the epiglottis comes into view the tip of the instrument passes posterior to it until the posterior larynx is visualised. It is important to keep to the midline as the left pyriform fossa may otherwise be entered.

Displacing the epiglottis anteriorly the vocal cords come to view.

The instrument is turned through 90° with the tip to the right and passed through the cords while turning the instrument into its neutral position. In order to follow the line of the trachea it is usual to lower the head-piece, otherwise the tip of the instrument would scrape the posterior tracheal wall.

Further inspection should present no problem.

The flexible bronchoscope can easily be introduced under light sedation and local anaesthesia. Because of its smaller size and flexibility it permits the examination of the distal bronchial tree, otherwise inaccessible to rigid bronchoscopy. Its disadvantage is that the view obtained is often inferior to the rigid bronchoscope due to mucus or blood covering the viewing lens. Because of the relatively small channel available, tenacious mucus and blood may be difficult to aspirate. The flexible

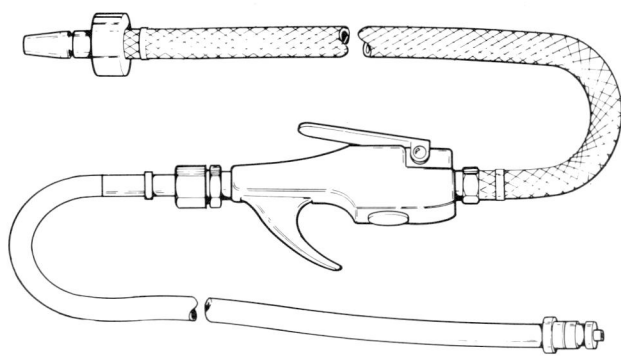

Fig.9 Venturi line

instrument also has a limited use in removal of foreign bodies.

From the above description it can be seen that rigid and flexible bronchoscopes are complementary and should be used as such.

Stradling, P. (1981) *Diagnostic Bronchoscopy*, 4th edn. Churchill Livingstone, Edinburgh.

Sanders, R.D. (1967) Two ventilating attachments for bronchoscopes. *Delaware Medical Journal*, **39**, 170.

Hetzel, M.R. (1982) New techniques: 3. Chest medicine. *Hospital Update*, Nov 1982, 1393-1402.

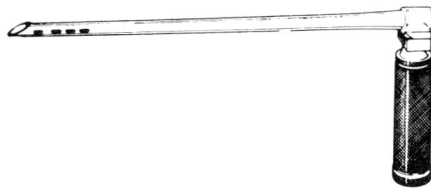

Fig.10 Emergency anaesthetic bronchoscope (Downs)

1.3 Mediastinoscope

Superior mediastinal lymph nodes are frequently involved in bronchial carcinoma. Examination and biopsy of these nodes can prevent unnecessary surgery. Prior to the introduction of mediastinoscopy a scalene node biopsy was employed to detect involvement of superior mediastinal nodes but this was shown to be inaccurate. Harken in 1954, aware of the shortcomings of scalene node biopsy, showed that it was possible to explore and examine the superior mediastinum by passing a laryngoscope into it through a scalene node biopsy incision. Although he achieved a higher diagnostic success it soon became apparent that this procedure was inaccurate, as it examined only one side of the mediastinum and contralateral spread of bronchial carcinoma is not infrequent. In 1959, Carlens described mediastinoscopy as we know it today.

The superior mediastinal nodes are divided into anterior mediastinal, tracheobronchial and paratracheal. Of these three groups the anterior mediastinal nodes lie in front of the ascending aorta and aortic arch, making them inaccessible to mediastinoscopy.

The procedure is performed under general anaesthesia and should be preceded by bronchoscopy. A transverse incision is made in the suprasternal notch and the pre-tracheal muscles are separated away from the midline. The pre-tracheal fascia is incised transversely and its lower flap reflected anteriorly. Using a finger, a tunnel is made between the fascia and trachea down to the carina, while the surrounding tissues are palpated for invasion and fixity. The finger then breaks the pre-tracheal fascia anterolaterally.

At this stage the mediastinoscope is inserted into the tunnel and the individual groups of lymph nodes are examined. Further blunt dissection is done under direct vision.

The mortality of this procedure is lower than that of exploratory thoracotomy.

The main complications include major haemorrhage, wound infection, recurrent laryngeal nerve damage and pneumothorax.

Harken, D.E., Black, H., Clauss R. and Ferrand, R.E. (1954) *New England Journal of Medicine*, **251**, 1071.
Carlens, E. (1959) *Diseases of the Chest*, **36**, 343.
Carlens, E. (1971) In: *Mediastinoscopy: Proceedings of an International Symposium* (ed. Jepsen, O. and Sorensen, H.R.). Odense University Press, Denmark.
Nohl-Oser, H.C. (1976) Mediastinoscopy. *British Journal of Hospital Medicine*, July 1976, 33-36.

1.4 Gastrointestinal endoscopy

Oesophagoscope

Examination of the oesophagus has become a standard part of gastroduodenoscopy.

The rigid oesophagoscope is now rarely used because it has few advantages over the flexible instrument and is more likely to cause perforation. However, it may be used to advantage for removal of foreign bodies and in therapeutic injection of oesophageal varices.

The rigid oesophagoscope of the Negus or Chevalier–Jackson pattern is a hollow tube, usually 45 cm long and 16–20 mm in diameter. It may be oval or circular in cross section. The differences between this instrument and the bronchoscope have been described in section 1.2. On its anterior aspect the instrument is calibrated in centimetres from the distal end. A rigid handle at right angles to the long axis is provided to facilitate insertion. Modern instruments are illuminated by fibrelight.

The procedure is carried out under endotracheal anaesthesia with the patient lying supine. A sandbag is placed behind the upper thoracic spine with the assistant holding the head.

With the neck fully flexed the instrument is guided over the operator's left hand over the tongue to the posterior pharyngeal wall. while the head is being extended the instrument is passed under direct vision behind the endotracheal tube until the cricopharyngeal fold comes to view. The instrument is advanced further until the head is fully extended.

The important anatomical constrictions are the crico-pharyngeal at 15 cm, the aortic and bronchial at 25 cm and the diaphragmatic at 40 cm. The procedure must be always carried out under direct vision without undue force, as perforation can readily take place. Flexible oesophagoscopy is discussed under flexible gastroduodenoscopy.

Gastroduodenoscope

Before the introduction of flexible fibreoptics the examination of the stomach and duodenum was mostly limited to barium studies. Semiflexible gastroscopes were introduced in the 1930s but never achieved popularity. The Japanese developed a blind gastrocamera in the 1950s but this too never caught on in clinical practice.

The situation changed with the introduction of flexible fibreoptics.

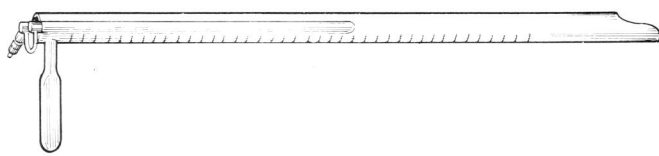

Fig.11 Negus oesophagoscope (Downs)

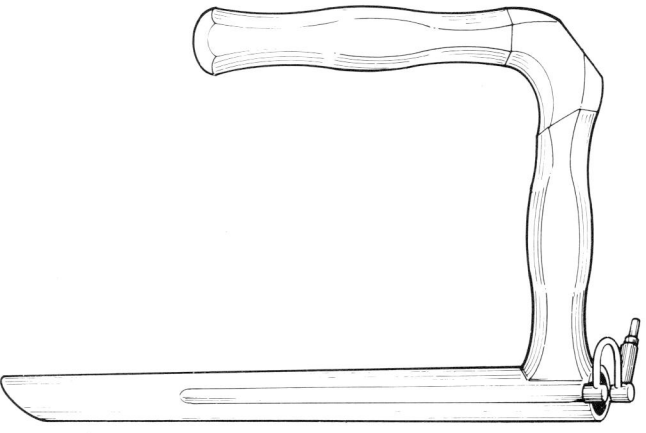

Fig.12 Negus oesophageal speculum (Downs)

The modern fibrescope consists of a head, with controls and eyepiece, and a flexible tube. The tip is manoeuvred by the head controls, and contains a viewing lens with a light source and air/water and biopsy/suction channels.

The optical system is a bundle 4 mm wide consisting of several thousand glass fibres. Each fibre is coated with glass of lower optical density, preventing light from leaking out. The fibres are spatially organised such that the optical image is composed of thousands of fine dots, and consequently the image quality cannot equal that of the rigid optical rod system.

At each end of the fibrescope is a lens system, adjustable at the proximal end and fixed at the tip. Light is transmitted from an external source via a cord through a separate bundle of fibres in the instrument. The external source of light is a halogen or arc lamp which is focused on to the bundle by a mirror. The intensity of light can be controlled by a system of filters and a diaphragm. The light source with its cooling system and the suction, air and water pumps are usually housed in one box.

Most instruments allow movement of the tip in two planes, at right angles to each other. The tip can be placed

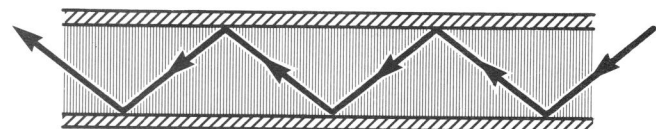

Fig.14 Principle of fibrelight transmission

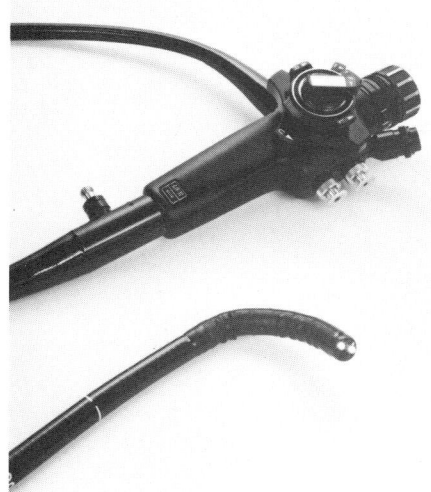

Fig.13 Olympus GIF-IT large channel therapeutic gastro-duodenoscope (Key Med)

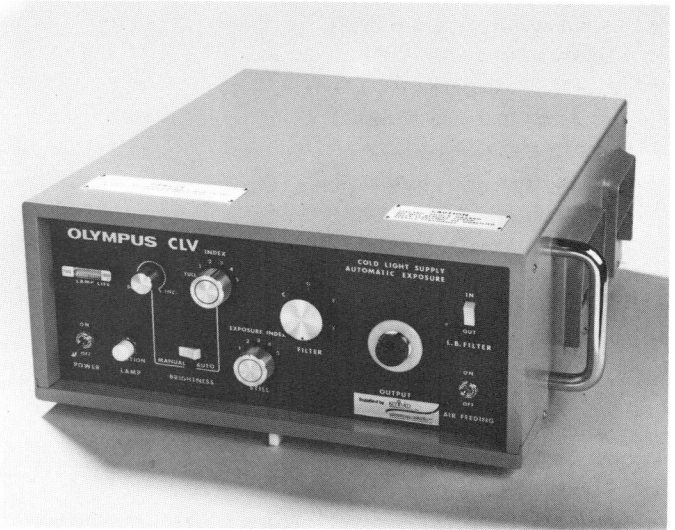

Fig.15 Olympus CLV high intensity light source, suitable for use with any Olympus flexible or rigid endoscope (Key Med)

10 DIAGNOSTIC INSTRUMENTS

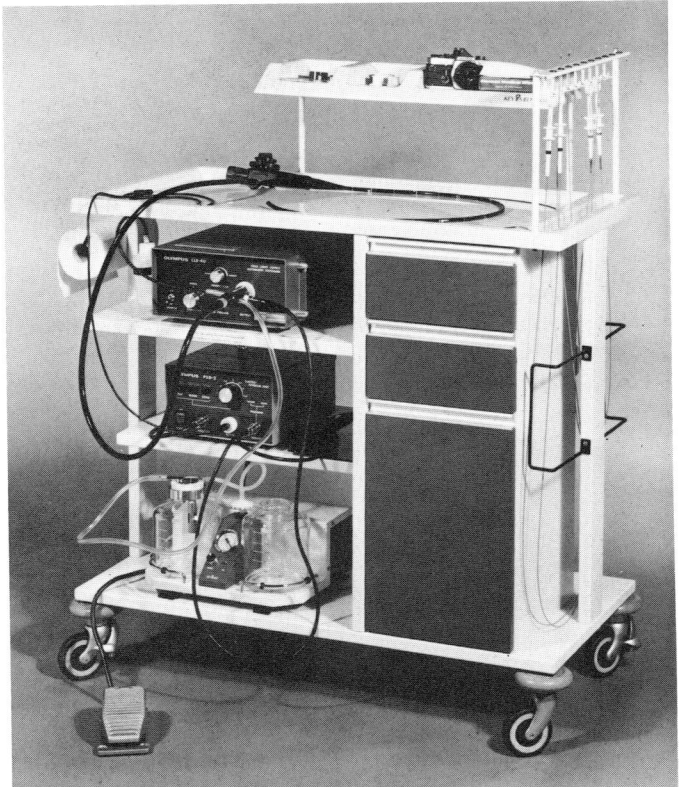

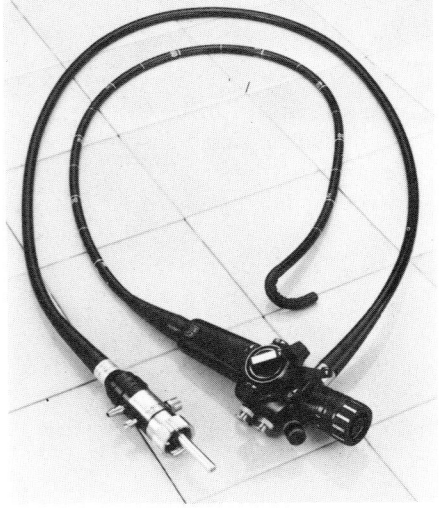

Fig.16 A Key Med endoscopy trolley prepared for a therapeutic gastro-duodenoscopy, complete with light source, suction pump and diathermy unit (Key Med)

Fig.17 Olympus GIF-XQ ultra slim oesophago-gastro-duodenoscope for diagnosis and therapy (Key Med)

beyond 180°. Movement is achieved by pull wires controlled by wheels in the handle. Each position can be locked in.

The viewing system can be arranged at the tip, to allow direct forward viewing, or at the side, for side viewing. The latter arrangement is necessary in some parts of the stomach and duodenum, especially for biopsy or instrumentation, as in the case of ERCP.

The smaller of the two channels provides air for inflation as well as a water jet which is squirted on to the lens. The larger channel is usually 2–3 mm in diameter and allows the passage of biopsy forceps, biopsy brushes and diathermy. It is also used for aspiration with an external suction pump.

Cotton, P.B. (1976) Upper gastrointestinal endoscopy. *British Journal of Hospital Medicine*, July 1976, 7-15.
Cotton, P.B. and Williams, C.B. (1982) *Practical Gastrointestinal Endoscopy*, 2nd edn. Blackwell Scientific Publications, Oxford.

OPTICAL INSTRUMENTS

Proctoscope

The proctoscope permits the examination of the lowermost part of the rectum and anus.

Unlike the sigmoidoscope it almost invariably has a handle. The anus has a tendency to push out the cone-shaped instrument and the handle is needed to maintain the instrument in position and for manipulation. There are numerous variations on the basic shape and some instruments may be more cone-shaped than others. Some operating proctoscopes may have a bevelled distal end or even a sliding removable segment.

Most proctoscopes are metal, but disposable plastic transparent proctoscopes are available. Because plastic is a poor heat conductor these instruments are particularly suitable for cryosurgery and diathermy.

The proctoscope is used mainly for diagnostic purposes and also for some minor therapeutic procedures, such as injection or banding of haemorrhoids, biopsy and local surgical procedures.

The instrument consists of a hollow cone-shaped tube with an obturator. The obturator obliterates the distal end of the proctoscope and the blunt end facilitates its insertion into the anus.

Fibrelight has now replaced the old-fashioned battery-powered bulb and provides excellent illumination. More expensive instruments have distal fibrelight illumination which is superior to the standard arrangement of proximal lighting source. It provides

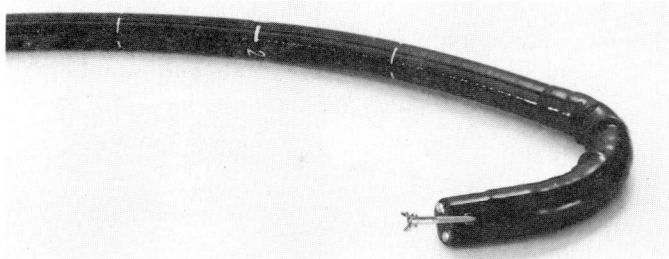

Fig.18 Distal tip of fore-oblique viewing Olympus GIF-K2 oesophago-gastroscope, ideal for injection of oesophageal varices. (Key Med)

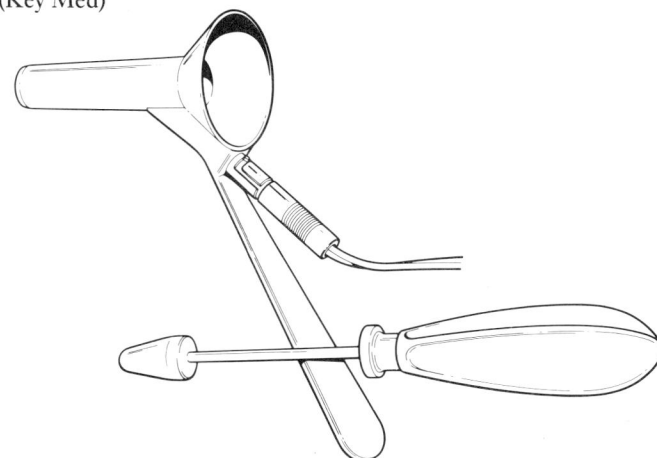

Fig.19 Naunton Morgan rectal speculum (Downs)

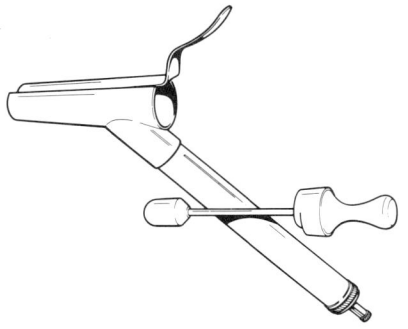

Fig.20 McEvedy rectal speculum (Downs)

unhindered access through the lumen, and faecal soiling reduces the amount of intra-luminal light very slightly.

Sigmoidoscope

The sigmoidoscope is in effect a rectoscope, since it rarely reaches the large bowel beyond the recto-sigmoid junction. Most rigid sigmoidoscopes are 25 cm long, but 30 cm, 20 cm and 15 cm lengths are not unusual. The standard external diameter is 20 cm and the narrower variety is usually preferable in the straightforward, unprepared and nervous patient.

The flexible sigmoidoscope is effectively a short colonoscope and will be discussed under that heading.

The standard sigmoidoscope, such as the Lloyd-Davies model, consists of a cylindrical tube with a removeable obturator, lighting system, closing window and double blower.

The modern sigmoidoscope has not changed very much over the years, except for its lighting system.

The previously inefficient and unreliable bulb and battery system has been replaced with a fibrelight which is either proximally or distally placed in the tube. The most efficient is the distal annular lighting system, which does not obstruct the lumen and provides good distal illumination even when soiled with faeces.

Sigmoidoscopy allows biopsy of lesions and mucosa and even removal of small polypoid tumours with a wire

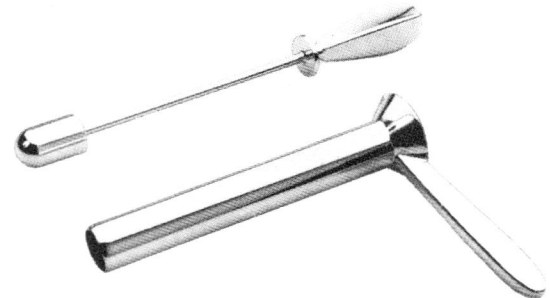

Fig.21 Kelly proctoscope (Downs)

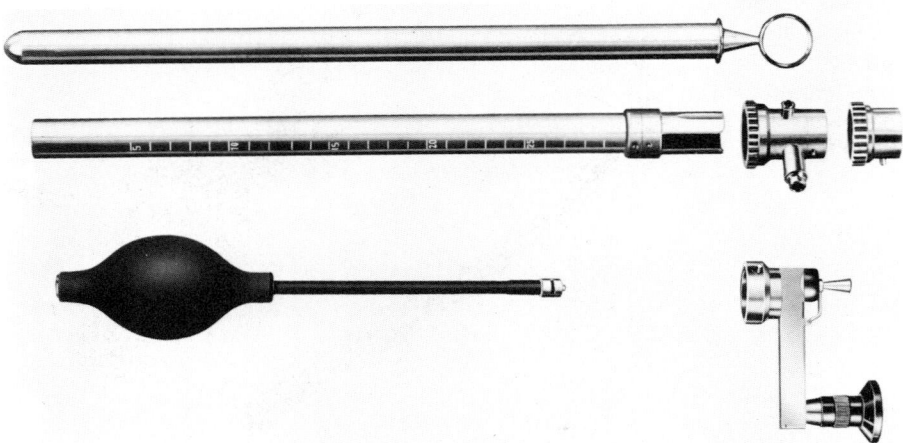

Fig.22 Heinkel sigmoidoscope (Storz)

snare. The insulated or plastic sigmoidoscopes may be used for cryosurgery or diathermy.

The best position for sigmoidoscopy, as well as for proctoscopy, is left lateral (Sims) position. A sandbag placed under the left buttock facilitates negotiation of lateral rectal curvatures.

The instrument is inserted with the obturator *in situ*. It is gently passed into the anus pointing towards the umbilicus. As soon as the rectum has been entered the obturator is removed and the lighting system with window and blower is attached.

Further passage of the instrument is done entirely under direct vision with gentle insufflation. As the rectum follows the sacral curve the instrument is appropriately angled.

The recto-sigmoid junction at 15 cm is difficult to negotiate in a large proportion of patients. Here the instrument needs to be angled dorsally and to the patient's right.

Lockhart-Mummery, H.E. (1976) *Operative Surgery* (ed. Robb, C. and Smith, R.). Butterworths, London.

Nicholls, R.J. (1982) Sigmoidoscopy. *British Journal of Hospital Medicine*, 56-66.

Vellacott, K.D. and Hardcastle, J.D. (1981) An evaluation of flexible fibreoptic sigmoidoscopy. *British Medical Journal*, **283**, 1583-1586.

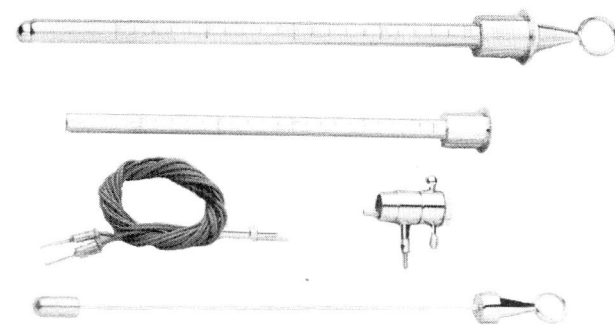

Colonoscope

Colonoscopy is supplementary to contrast studies and rigid proctosigmoidoscopy and should be considered as a second-line procedure in most cases. However, in certain situations, such as bleeding, polyposis and long-standing ulcerative colitis, colonoscopy may be considered as a front-line procedure.

Fig.23 Lloyd Davies sigmoidoscope (Downs)

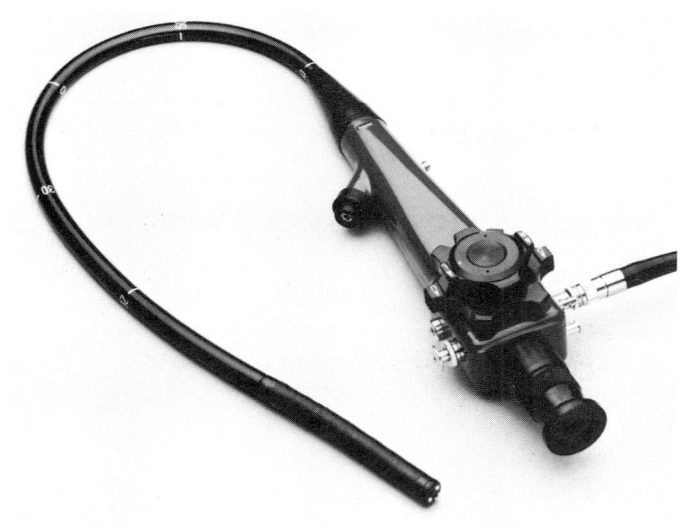

Fig.24 Olympus OSF out-patient flexible sigmoidoscope (Key Med)

The colonoscope is a more robust instrument than other flexible endoscopes. It is thicker and is available in several lengths. Long colonoscopes measure up to 180 cm in length and are designed to reach the caecum. The medium instruments are 130–140 cm and in most cases should reach the caecum. The shortest instruments (70–110 cm) are in fact sigmoidoscopes.

The longer the instrument, the more easily it becomes damaged, and so its fibres need replacing at more frequent intervals. The cost is also directly proportional to the instrument's length. The controls, fibreoptics and accessory channels are the same as in gastroduodenoscopes.

Williams, C.B. (1976) Colonoscopy. In: *Operative Surgery* (ed. Robb, C. and Smith, R.). Butterworths, London.
Cotton, P.B. and Williams, C.B. (1982) *Practical Gastrointestinal Endoscopy*, 2nd edn. Blackwell Scientific Publications, Oxford.

1.5 Choledoschoscope

Choledoschoscopy is the technique of visualisation of the common and hepatic bile ducts through choledochotomy. The use of peroperative cholangiography and standard bile duct exploration has inherent problems and may lead to retention of stones or failure to diagnose bile duct neoplasm. The choledoschoscope has been introduced to improve diagnostic accuracy of bile duct exploration.

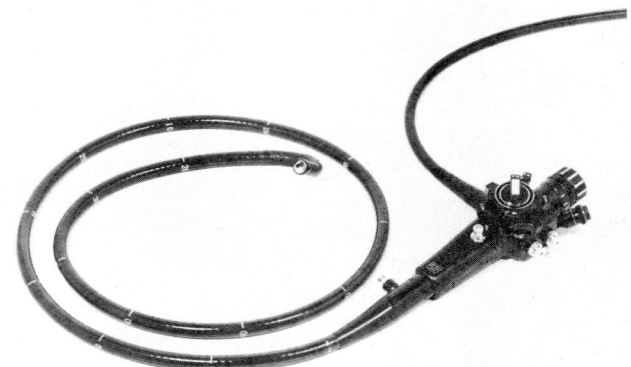

Fig.25 Olympus CF-ITL large channel colonofiberscope for total therapeutic colonoscopy (Key Med)

The rigid choledochoscope is an L-shaped instrument which incorporates lighting, viewing and irrigating systems. Two sizes are available, with identical vertical limbs, and with a horizontal limb either 40 or 60 mm long.

The lighting and optical systems are of the Hopkins design.

Saline is used for irrigation.

Instrument channels, allowing the use of biopsy forceps, Fogarty catheter, Dormia basket and a biopsy brush, are detachable.

The instrument is sterilised in ethylene oxide gas.

The standard choledochotomy incision allows the introduction of the

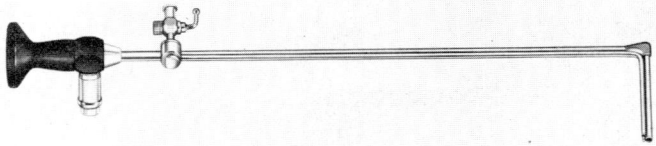

Fig.26 Choledochoscope (Storz)

instrument, which is 5×3 mm in diameter.

The instrument is first inserted towards the ampulla and is advanced further under direct vision until the sphincter opening of the common bile duct is seen.

The instrument is then withdrawn, rotated by 180° and reinserted through choledochotomy to visualise the hepatic ducts.

Recently, flexible choledochoscopes have been introduced but these are very delicate, expensive instruments, and because of a small irrigation channel, limited instrumentation is possible.

Benci, G., Shore, M.J., Morgenstern, L. and Hamlin, J.A. (1978) Choledochoscopy and operative fluorocholangiography in the prevention of retained bile duct stones. *World Journal of Surgery*, **2**, 411-427.

1.6 Laparoscope

The first purpose-built laparoscope was used in 1929 by Kalk, although examination of the peritoneal cavity with a cytoscope was reported as early as 1902 by Kelling. Since then laparoscopy has been used extensively, mainly by gynaecologists, not only for the examination of the pelvis but also for some therapeutic procedures such as tubal ligation.

More recently, general surgeons and gastroenterologists have shown interest in this diagnostic tool as an alternative to laparotomy and to facilitate biopsy from specific organs.

This procedure is performed under general anaesthetic although local or regional anaesthesia with sedation may be used.

The basic laparoscopy set consists of an automatic gas insufflator, Verres cannula, trochar and telescope with a light source.

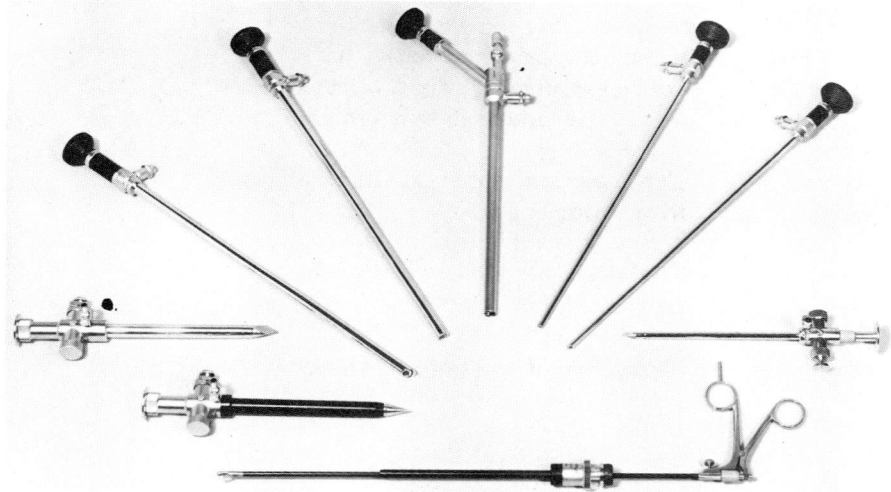

Fig.27 A range of Olympus laproscopes and accessories (Key Med)

Carbon dioxide is most commonly used for insufflation of the peritoneum. Air should not be used and nitrous oxide is contraindicated with the use of diathermy. Nitrous oxide, however, causes less discomfort to the patient, presumably due to its anaesthetic effect.

Gas is introduced into the peritoneal cavity via a Verres needle which is inserted through the linea alba just below the umbilicus. The needle has a spring-loaded blunt stylet. When the distal blunt point is pushed against the linea alba or peritoneum it is pushed inside the lumen thus allowing the outer sharp needle to penetrate these layers. As soon as these layers have been pierced the point springs back, thus minimising the risk of damaging viscus.

The gas insufflator registers flow rate and intraperitoneal pressure. The flow rate should be approximately 0.5 $l.m^{-1}$ and the intraperitoneal pressure should not exceed 20 cm of water. The total volume of gas insufflated varies between 2 and 4 litres.

The Verres needle is then withdrawn and, the trochar is inserted through a small incision, and directed obliquely towards the pelvis to avoid major blood vessels. The trochar obturator is withdrawn and a spring-loaded valve prevents the escape of gas. The trochar is then replaced with a viewing or operating telescope. Modern telescopes have the Hopkins rod-lens system which apart from improved light transmission and

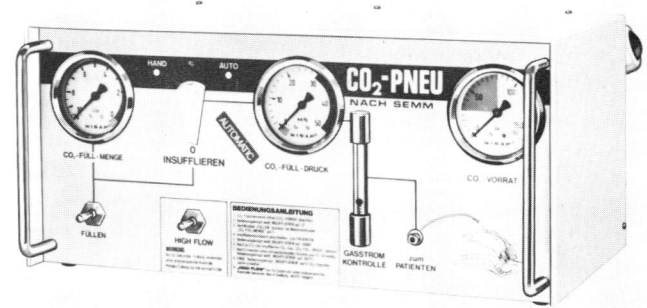

Fig.28 Automatic gas insufflator (Storz)

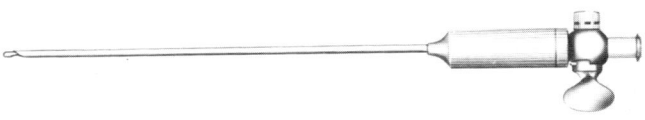

Fig.29 Verres cannula (Storz)

resolution and a brighter image has a wider viewing angle. A manipulating probe may be inserted at a site distant from the entry of the laparoscope to allow manipulation of tissues.

At the end of the procedure the obturator valve is opened allowing gas to escape; the obturator is removed and the wound closed. The contraindications for this procedure are cardiac insufficiency, internal or external abdominal herniae, abdominal wall or peritoneal sepsis and haemorrhagic diathesis. Known peritoneal adhesions and extensive scarring of the abdominal wall make the procedure hazardous. The procedure has the complications of any major surgical intervention. The specific complications include gas embolism, visceral injury and subcutaneous emphysema.

Kalk, H. (1929) Erfarurgen mit der Laparoskopie. *Zeitschrift für Klinische Medizine*, 111, 303.

Matheson, N.A. (1976) Diagnostic laparoscopy. In: *Operative Surgery* (ed. Robb, C. and Smith, R.). Butterworths, London.

Cuschieri, A. (1980) Laparoscopy in general surgery and gastroenterology. *British Journal of Hospital Medicine*, September 1980, 252.

1.7 Arthroscope

Arthroscopy is an endoscopic examination of joints and has clear advantages over exploratory arthrotomy in terms of lower risk of infection and morbidity. The knee joint is the most accessible for this examination.

Although knee arthroscopy was first carried out as early at 1918 by Takagi, it has been used increasingly since the 1950s.

Knee arthroscopy is indicated for a variety of injuries and chronic conditions of the knee, such as chondromalacia patellae, osteochondritis dissecans and arthritis.

The arthroscope is a rigid instrument consisting of a steel sheath, trochars and telescopes. The sheath is attached to an irrigating system and is 5 mm in diameter. If biopsy forceps are used, the standard 4 mm telescope is replaced with a 2.7 mm telescope to accommodate both within the sheath. As in other rigid endoscopic instruments the telescopes have a varied angle of view.

If carried out under general anaesthesia the leg is exsanguinated by elevation and Esmarch bandage, with a pneumatic tourniquet applied to the thigh.

With the knee flexed a small incision is made 1 cm medial to the patellar tendon, approximately 1 cm below the inferior border of the patella.

The sheath with a trochar is introduced through the incision into the joint space, pointing laterally, behind the ligamentum patellae, just above the lateral meniscus. The sharp trochar is then replaced with a blunt trochar, and with the knee extended the sheath is inserted into the suprapatellar pouch. The tochar is removed and replaced with the telescope, attached to the sheath by a bridge. The cold light source with irrigation system is then connected.

The joint is distended with saline and both inflow and outflow taps closed.

Alternatively, the joint may be distended via a separate intra-articular needle prior to the introduction of the instrument.

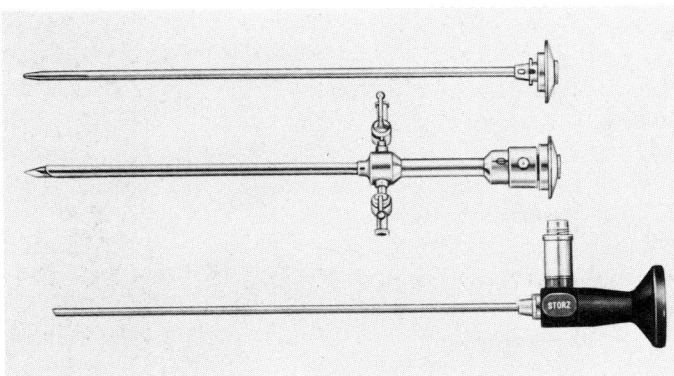

Fig.30 Arthroscope (Storz)

18 DIAGNOSTIC INSTRUMENTS

The knee joint is now ready for the examination. At the end of the examination the joint is emptied of fluid and the instrument is withdrawn.

The wound is closed with sutures and a compression bandage applied.

Bentley, G. and Leslie, I.J. (1976) Arthroscopy of the knee. In: *Operative Surgery* (ed. Robb, C. and Smith, R.). Butterworths, London

Jackson, R.W. and Dandy, D.J. (1976) *Arthroscopy of the Knee*. Grune & Stratton, New York.

1.8 Urological endoscopy

Cysto-urethroscope

The cysto-urethroscope is the very basis of urological diagnostic tools. It is designed to allow visualisation of the urethra and urinary bladder.

The operating cystoscope has a facility for catheterisation of strictures and ureters, biopsy and diathermy. The first cystoscope was developed by Nitze in 1876. By 1880 a lens telescope and electric lighting systems were added. Initially, the cystoscope was a one-piece instrument but later the lighting and viewing telescope became detachable, to allow bladder irrigation.

The cysto-urethroscope consists of an outer sheath and a telescope with a lens system and light source. The sheath is a metal tube, oval in cross section, commonly of 19 or 23.5 FG size.

The end is slightly curved to allow for the natural curve of the male

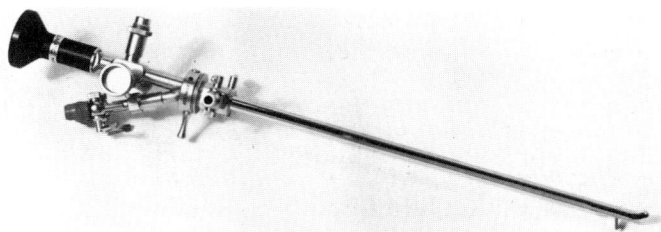

Fig.31 Olympus adult cystoscope (Key Med)

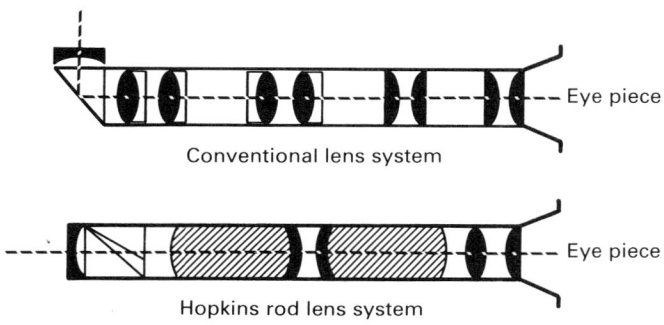

Fig.32 Principle of bulb-lit and fibre-lit telescopes

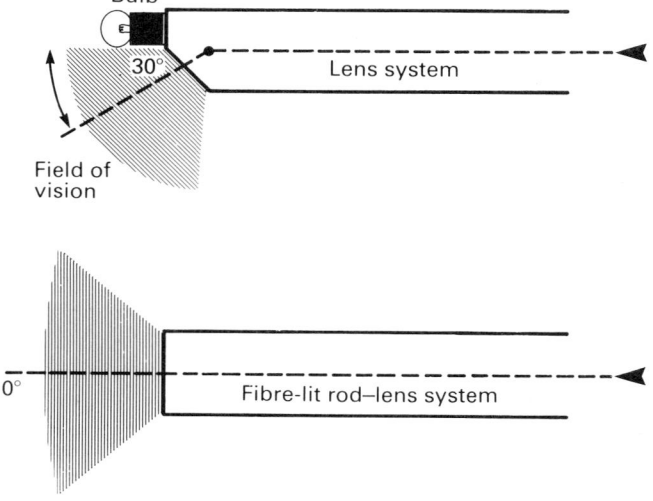

Fig.33 Principle of conventional and Hopkins rod-lens telescopes

urethra. An obturator provides a blunt end for insertion into the bladder. At the proximal end is an attachment lock for accessories.

Two valves are provided for inlet and outlet of irrigating fluid. The viewing and lighting systems are incorporated in the telescope.

Prior to the introduction of fibre lighting, telescopes were lit by electric bulbs. The disadvantage of this was that illumination was poor and unreliable, and direct viewing was impossible, due to the interfering light bulb.

Although the possibility of transmission of light through a glass fibre was first demonstrated in 1927 by Baird, it was Hopkins in 1954 who applied its principle to his rod-lens optical system. By coating a glass rod with a coat of glass of different refractive index, light entering one end of the rod will be transmitted to the other end by internal reflection. Very thin fibres in bundles are flexible and form the basis of flexible light-conducting cables.

Before the introduction of Hopkins' rod lens system, the viewing telescope consisted of an eyepiece, transmitting lenses and an objective lens. The disadvantage of this system was lack of detail, especially in the periphery of the field, and poor light transmission.

The Hopkins system makes use of solid glass rods with fixed lenses which replace the air spaces. The small air spaces between the rods serve as air lenses, with the result that twice the amount of light is transmitted for a given diameter. The rods can be made and adjusted with greater accuracy, resulting in better resolution of the image. The angle of view is twice as large as that of the conventional lens system — approximately 70°.

Telescopes are made with four standard axes of view: Straight forward 0°, forward-oblique 30°, lateral 70°, and retrospective telescope 120°.

Blandy, J. (1978) *Transurethral Resection.* 2nd edn. Pitman Medical, London.
Gow, J.G. (1976) Urological technology.

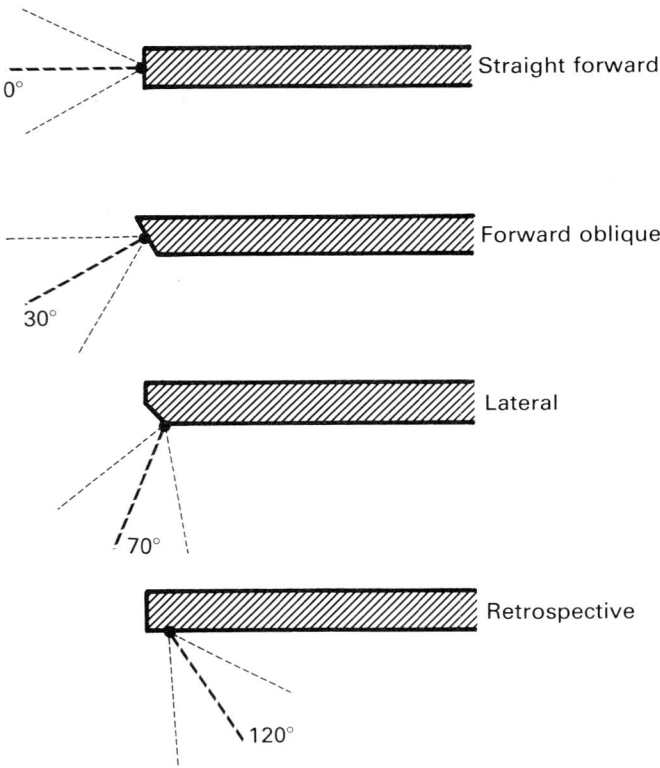

Fig.34 Diagram of straight forward, forward, lateral and retrospective telescopes

In: *Urology 1* (ed. Blandy, J.). Blackwell Scientific Publications, Oxford.

Hopkins, H.H. and Kapany, N.S. (1954) A flexible fibrescope using static scanning. *Nature, Lond.*, **173**, 39.

Ureteroscope

The rigid ureteroscope is a recent addition to the urologist's armament. Ureteroscopy is less invasive than percutaneous nephroscopy, and in a large proportion of patients the renal pelvis can be visualised. Although flexible ureteroscopes have been available for some time, these have many disadvantages: high cost and considerable fragility, poor quality of visual image and small size of the operating channel. The instrument is essentially a long, thin cystoscope. It is 50 cm in length and the sheath size is 11 FG, although 9 FG is also available.

As with a conventional cystoscope, the ureteroscope has an irrigating system and an operating channel for biopsy, brush cytology or Dormia instrumentation. The optical system is 0° or 70°.

Prior to the insertion of the ureteroscope, the ureteric orifice can be dilated with a ureteric probe up to the size of the ureteroscope sheath. This manoeuvre is essential because the passage through the intramural ureter represents the most difficult part of the procedure. The instrument is then inserted into the bladder in the conventional way and then, after visualisation of the ureteric orifice, into the ureter.

The irrigation pressure should be low (30–40 cm H_2O) to avoid over-distension.

No serious injuries have been reported but ureteric perforation is possible.

Perez-Castro Ellendt, E. and Martinez-Pineiro, J.A. (1982) *European Urology*, **8**, 117-120.

Nephroscope

Nephroscopy is the technique of visualisation of the renal pelvis and calyces through an incision in the renal pelvis.

Percutaneous nephroscopy is discussed in Chapter 11.

The technique and instrument for operative nephroscopy are the same as for the choledochoscope.

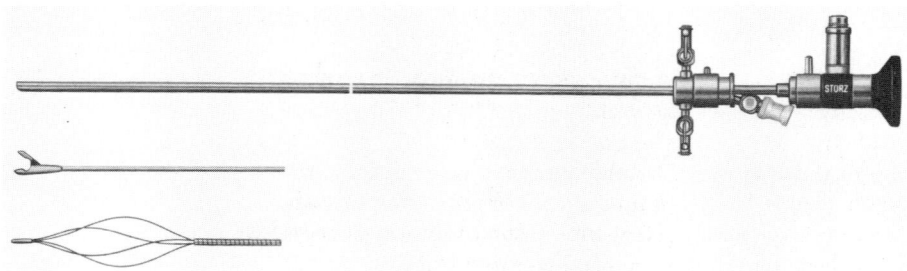

Fig.35 Ureteroscope (Storz)

Chapter 2

Ultrasound, Image Intensifier, CT Scan, Urodynamics

2.1 Diagnostic ultrasound
2.2 Image intensifier
2.3 Computerised axial tomography
2.4 Urodynamics

2.1 Diagnostic ultrasound

Ultrasound is a mechanical vibration at a frequency beyond the hearing threshold of the human ear (20 000 Hz). The production and detection of ultrasound is based on the observation by Jacques and Pierre Curie in 1880 that compression of a quartz crystal produces an alternation of charge across it — the piezoelectric effect. When current is applied the crystal deforms at a frequency directly related to the voltage applied, producing ultrasound. Equally, the same crystal, exposed to ultrasound, wil produce a voltage change — the converse piezoelectric effect.

Modern ultrasound utilises artificial materials, the polarised polycrystalline ferroelectrics such as calcium barium titanate or lead zirconium titanate. In medical diagnosis, ultrasound is generated by applying voltage to a transducer disc, resulting in resonation. The thinner the disc, the higher is the frequency of ultrasound generated.

To produce a directional beam of ultrasound the transducer is placed at one end of a hollow tube, the probe. The ultrasound produced from the opposite surface of the transducer is damped down by a suitable material. The probe also serves as a receiver for the returning ultrasound echos. These produce voltage changes in the transducer which are amplified and reproduced on a cathode-ray oscilloscope.

There are two basic ultrasonic diagnostic techniques: the pulse echo and the Doppler effect. The pulse technique generates 500–1000 ultrasound pulses per second. Between pulses the transducer records the returning ultrasound echo. In A-scan technique display, the echoes are recorded as vertical deflections on the cathode-ray oscilloscope. Echoes arising from the skin are displayed on the left-hand side of the screen and the echoes from underlying organs are displayed to the right in direct proportion to their distance from the skin. The height of each deflection by each echo is proportional to its strength.

Brightness modulation display, also known as B-scan, records echoes as bright dots along the baseline of the oscilloscope. The baseline follows the direction of the ultrasound beam, and as the probe is moved along the skin the dots build up a picture of the tissues under the probe.

Time-position (M-mode) display is developed from the B-scan and is used for display of moving structures such as the heart. The echo dots from the moving organ are swept by a slow-speed time-base generator, thus producing a moving picture which can be photographed or recorded on a running strip of photographic paper. Real-time display ultrasound provides a moving picture by producing sequential ultrasound pictures at a speed of 40 per second. These displays are not truly instantaneous since they are delayed by the time interval between each picture and the varying depth of structures exposed to the beam. The main limitation of diagnostic ultrasound is its inability to pass through gases and therefore it has a limited use in the thorax and abdomen. It is also time consuming and requires considerable expertise. Its advantage lies in non-invasiveness, safety and the ability to differentiate between solid masses and cysts.

The Doppler effect ultrasound is based on the observations of Christian Doppler, who in 1843 described the sound frequency change when a sound moves towards or away from a stationary observer.

In 1959 Satomura described the application of the Doppler effect to detection of the blood flow. The ultrasound wave is reflected by erythrocytes moving in a blood vessel and is detected by another transducer. The outgoing signal is subtracted from the echo to produce an audible sound. The sound so produced is dependent on the velocity of erythrocytes within the blood stream under the ultrasound beam. The frequency shift between the emitted and reflected signals is called the Doppler shift. Providing that the ultrasound frequency and its velocity in tissues are constant, the shift is directly proportional to the velocity of erythrocytes and the angle between the beam and the blood vessel. Flow in a given vessel cannot be estimated by this technique if used non-invasively, because of the size of the vessel and the angle are unknown. Thus the simplest Doppler probes are able to detect blood movement only. Direction Doppler is capable of detecting the direction of blood flow by introducing a 90° phase shift into the echo which is added or subtracted from the Doppler shift depending on the direction of the flow.

The ultrasonic frequencies used depend on the depth of the vessel under study; higher frequencies are used for superficial vessels and lower frequencies for deeper vessels. Most Doppler probes produce continuous wave ultrasound and therefore contain two piezoelectric crystals, one emitting and the other receiving.

Pulsed Dopplers are capable of detecting returning signals from tissues under examination, while ignoring other signals entering the probe.

Dear, A.R. and Lumley, J.S.P. (1981) Ultrasonic assessment of vascular disorders. In: *Surgical Review 2* (ed. Lumley, J.S.P. and Craven, JL), p. 369. Pitman Medical, London.

Satomura, S. (1959) Study of flow patterns in peripheral arteries by ultrasonics. *Journal of Acoustic Science of Japan*, 15, 151.

McLeod, F.D. (1967) A directional Doppler flowmeter. *Proceeding of the Annual Conference on Engineering in Medicine and Biology*, 9, 27.

McDicken, W.N. (1976) *Diagnostic Ultrasonics: Principles and Use of Instruments*. Crosby, Lockwood & Staples, London.

Ross, F. (1980) Ultrasound (1) Principles:

General: Cardiac. In: *A Textbook of Radiology and Imaging* (ed. Sutton, D.), 3rd edn, p. 1339. Churchill Livingstone, Edinburgh.

2.2 Image intensifier

The image intensifier is increasingly used by surgeons in operating theatres for a variety of surgical procedures and some understanding of its principles is desirable.

An X-ray beam having passed through the patient's body can be made visible by allowing it to fall on to either a photographic film or a fluorescent screen. The development of photographic film will produce a negative picture. The effect of an X-ray beam on the fluorescent screen is to produce an emission of visible light photons in amount proportional to the incident X-ray intensity. The picture is visible as long as the beam is switched on. This technique is called fluoroscopy. Fluoroscopy has the advantage of being cheap compared to radiography in that it uses no film and processing chemicals and provides an immediate dynamic picture. However the brightness of fluoroscopic screen can be increased with reduced exposure by means of an image intensifier. The image can be observed either directly by means of a mirror system or via a television monitor.

The image intensifier provides a picture sufficiently bright to obviate the need for a darkened room. It consists of a fluorescent screen on which the X-ray beam is directed and a second screen, the photocathode, which is in close contact with the fluorescent screen.

The photocathode is composed of a photo-electron-emitting material and these emitted electrons will correspond in intensity to the pattern of light upon it. The electrons are accelerated across a vacuum tube by voltage applied between the photocathode and the fluorescent viewing screen. Due to the increased energy of electrons, the light on the output screen is very much brighter.

The surface of the output screen nearest to the photocathode is covered by a thin layer of aluminium which allows the electrons to pass through but prevents any light that is produced on the screen passing back to the photocathode. The electron lens reduces the size of the image to about one-fifth of the image on the fluorescent screen. In the absence of electron acceleration this leads to an increase in brightness by a factor of 25, since the same amount of energy is being passed through a smaller area. This reduction in size of the image can be compensated for by a magnifying optical system.

The increase in brightness because of electron acceleration is approximately fortyfold, so that the overall brightness is increased a thousandfold. The advantage of the image intensifier is that by reducing brightness less X-ray exposure is necessary. A reduction in patient dose by a factor of 10 will lead to an increase of brightness of one hundredfold — quite sufficient for normal vision. With increased brightness, perception of detail is greater, but even with modern screens blurring of the image occurs. One of the major defects of the image intensifier is the relatively small area that can be visualised at any time. The disadvantages of eyepiece viewing have been overcome by the use of a closed-circuit television.

The television screen also has the advantage that the brightness of the picture can be as great as required, irrespective of the input screen brightness, and this can lead to a further reduction in patient X-ray exposure.

2.3 Computerised axial tomography

Computerised axial tomography provides information about tissue density in a thin section of tissue. This revolutionary imaging technique was developed in 1972 by N. Hounsfield, for which he received a joint Nobel Prize for Medicine in 1979. The idea was based on the assumption that measurement of X-rays passing through the body could provide information on all tissues in the path of an X-ray beam and, when the beam is multidirectional, the data thus obtained could be computed and presented in a conventional form to produce a three-dimentional picture.

The X-ray beam is collimated to a narrow beam which passes through the body and is partially absorbed. The unabsorbed photons fall on to scintillation or ionization detectors. These detectors measure the number of photons, which is related to the density of tissues; the greater the tissue density the more photons are absorbed by it.

The data are quantified and processed by a computer. The X-ray beam is then rotated around the body in the same transverse plane and multiple readings are obtained. It is usual to present the readings in an analogue form on a screen in two dimensions. Here, each reading is represented by a single picture element, or pixel. The smaller each pixel, the greater is the number of pixels that can be accommodated on the screen and the better is the resolution of the picture. The screen presentation is in the form of Grayscale. The whiteness of tissue is proportional to the degree of X-ray beam attenuation at each point. Thus radiodense tissues appear white, and radiolucent tissues appear black.

The Hounsfield scale provides numerical values of tissue density relative to water (0) and air (-1000). Bone, for example, has a numerical value of $+100$ and fat -100.

The thickness of each section is determined by collimation of the beam and is $2-13$ mm thick. The early scanners used a simple collimated X-ray beam and scanning detectors which were rotated at $1°$ intervals over an arc of $180°$. This technique was time consuming and modern scanners employ collimated fan beams and a ring of detectors. The beam rotates either inside or outside the ring, thus shortening the scanning time to less than 20 seconds per section.

Housnfield, G.N. (1973) Computerised transverse axial scanning (tomography) — Part I: Description of system. *British Journal of Radiology*, **46**, 1016-1022.

Brooks, R.A., and Di Chiro, G. (1976) Principles of computer assisted tomography (CAT) in radiographic and radio-isotope imaging. *Physics in Medicine and Biology*, **21**, 689-732.

Moseley, I. and Sutton, D. (1980) CT scanning. In: *Textbook of Radiology and Imaging* (ed. Sutton, D.), 3rd edn, p. 1230. Churchill Livingstone, Edinburgh.

2.4 Urodynamics

Urodynamic investigation is a study of physiological changes that take place in disorders of the lower urinary tract. The procedure has its inherent limitations and the results have to be interpreted in the light of other investigations.

Urodynamic investigation is indicated in patients with persistent symptoms of the lower urinary tract when basic investigations, such as IVP and cystoscopy, failed to make a diagnosis. The measurement consists of four separate components: urethral profile, cystometrogram, pressure flow study and the optional voiding cystourethrography.

The investigation attempts to answer the following:
(1) the presence or absence of sphincter mechanism and whether it is under voluntary control;
(2) the presence or absence of outflow obstruction and its cause;
(3) sphincter dynamics;
(4) bladder capacity;
(5) detrusor contraction, whether involuntary or voluntary;
(6) sensation of the bladder.

A urethral pressure profile is a recording of pressure within and along the whole length of the urethra. The pressure is measured using a special cannula, closed at one end, with side holes 5 cm from this end. Fluid is infused through the cannula until an equilibrium is reached when the fluid within the cannula is under the same pressure as the outside pressure.

As the cannula is being withdrawn, the pressure changes that occur along the urethra are recorded on graph paper. Abnormalities such a bladder neck obstruction, absent external sphincter or urethral strictures can thus be shown.

Cystometry is a recording of bladder pressure changes in relation to volume. The bladder is filled with fluid and pressure changes within the bladder are recorded using a pressure transducer placed inside it. In order to subtract any pressure changes outside the bladder itself a rectal pressure balloon is inserted. The patient is asked to report the first sensation of bladder filling and when he feels a strong desire to void. The last sensation is taken as the bladder capacity.

Having removed the inflow catheter, the patient is asked to void and the presence of voluntary detrusor contraction is recorded. If involuntary detrusor contractions are suspected they can be provoked by manoeuvres such as coughing, supra-pubic tapping or positional changes.

The pressure flow is measured with a pressure transducer within the bladder while recording the flow rate during voiding. Quite a large proportion of patients are unable to void spontaneously. This recording measures the maximum flow, average flow and shape of the curve, and may reveal abdominal straining, unsustained bladder contractions or bladder outlet obstruction.

Voiding cystourethrography is a fluoroscopic recording of the lower urinary tract during bladder filling and voiding. It can pinpoint site of outflow obstruction, incompetent sphincter or even vesicoureteric reflux.

Blivas, J.G., Amad, S.A., Bissada, N., Khanna, O.P., Krane, R.J., Wein, A.J. and Yalla, S. (1982) Urodynamic procedures. Recommendations of the Urodynamic Society. I. Procedures that should be available for routine urologic practice. *Neurourology and Urodynamics*, **1**, 51-55.

Edwards, L.E. (1974) The urethral pressure profile. In: *The Diagnosis of Disorders of Micturition in Children* (ed. Johnson, J.H. and Goodwins, W.E.). *Reviews in Paediatric Urology*, 433-476.

Edwards, L.E. (1976) Incontinence of urine. In: *Urology II* (ed. Blandy, J.S.), p. 687. Blackwell Scientific Publications, Oxford

Chapter 3   Biopsies

3.1 Curette
3.2 Brush biopsy
3.3 Needle biopsy
3.4 Biopsy punch forceps
3.5 Trephine biopsy
3.6 High-speed drill biopsy
3.7 Diathermy snare and loop
3.8 Crosby–Kugler intestinal biopsy
3.9 Crybiopsy

Although macroscopic examination of organs or tissues is important, the final tissue diagnosis is made by histological examination of such tissues. Biopsy, within its limitations, is diagnostic.

Biopsy is defined as examination of living tissue removed from the body. For most of us it implies the act of removing a sample of tissue or, used as a noun, the piece of tissue removed.

The most direct way of taking a biopsy is to cut away a piece of tissue with a scalpel under direct vision. However, this is a formal operation, often requiring anaesthesia, and incision results in a scar. It has the advantage that the whole lump can be excised (excision biopsy) or a sizable part of it (incisional biopsy).

Cytology is a form of microscopical biopsy. The washing out or scraping of cells by artificial means involves removal of living or dead cells for examination.

There are numerous ways of taking a biopsy and all have their advantages and disadvantages. Most of them are described in this chapter.

3.1 Curette

The curette is a scoop-like instrument. It is used to scrape off material or tissue either for biopsy or as a part of debridement. Volkmann's spoon is the classical example of this instrument. It has a scoop of different sizes and shapes but in the original instrument this was circular. Currently used curettes have scoops at each end. The edges of the scoop are sharpened to facilitate scraping. Some curettes, such as the endometrial curette, have a fenestrated scoop, thus preventing tissue from accumulating. Curetting is particularly suitable for biopsy of cavities, ulcers or sinuses.

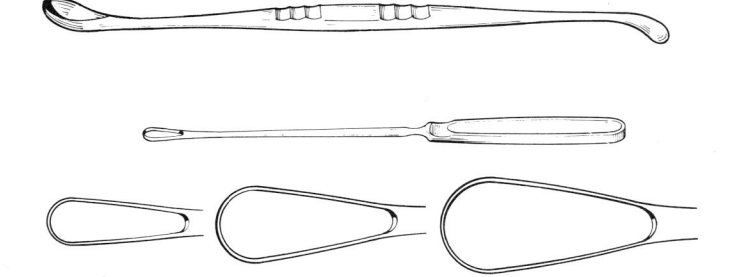

Fig.36 Volkmann scoop (Downs)

Fig.37 Sims uterine curette (Downs)

3.2 Brush biopsy

Brush biopsy does not remove a whole piece of tissue; rather it removes clumps of cells by virtue of its abrasive action. In effect, it is a cytological biopsy. It came to use with the introduction of flexible fibreoptic endoscopy.

The biopsy material is smeared onto a glass slide and immersed in a fixative prior to staining. The advantage of this technique is that it is less traumatic than formal punch biopsy and large areas of suspicious mucosa can be sampled. Its disadvantage is that interpretation of the biopsy material requires an experienced cytologist and, since the biopsy includes only the superficial layer of cells, deeper submucosal lesions may be missed. Although it has been used mainly in the upper gastrointestinal endoscopy it can be useful in the biliary and renal tracts as well as in the colon.

Villardell F. (1971) Exfoliative cytology of the oesophagus. *Digestion*, **4**, 59

Gephart, T. and Graham, R.M. (1959) The cellular detection of carcinoma of the oesophagus. *Surgery, Gynecology and Obstetrics*, **108**, 75

3.3 Needle biopsy

Needle biopsy is perhaps the most frequently used technique of biopsy, owing to its simplicity and speed. It is used for biopsy of superficial as well as deep tissues. The main advantage of this technique is that it can be performed under local anaesthesia with minimal facilities and a minimum of trauma.

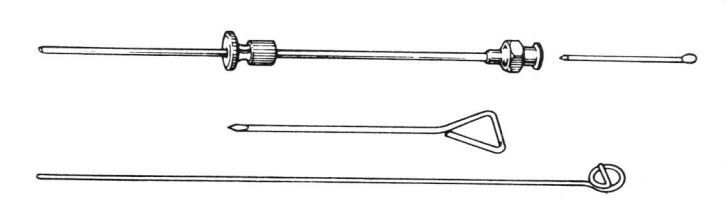

The size of the specimen obtained depends on the size and type of needle as well as on the operator's skill.

There are two basic types of biopsy needle: aspiration and cutting. The simplest aspiration biopsy can be carried out with a medium-size hypodermic needle attached to a syringe. By inserting the needle into a lesion, such as a breast lump, while exerting suction on the syringe, sufficient numbers of cells can be aspirated for diagnostic cytology. The Menghini needle is an aspiration-type biopsy needle which removes a cylinder of tissue approximately 1 mm in diameter, if the standard size is used. Its outside diameter is 1–1.9 mm. The needle consists of the needle sheath with a bevelled tip and a Luer-type attachment for the syringe. A blocking pin fits loosely into the proximal end of the needle and a stilette obstructs the lumen during its insertion. A guard may be fitted to the needle to prevent excessive penetration. The needle is connected to a 10 ml syringe containing several millilitres of saline. It is then inserted through tissues towards the organ or tissue to be biopsied and a small volume of saline is injected to clear

Fig.38 Menghini needle (Downs)

skin or debris from the needle lumen. Suction is then applied to the syringe, and the needle is thrust in and completely withdrawn. The specimen is removed by expressing the remaining saline in the syringe. The blocking pin prevents the biopsy being aspirated into the syringe lumen.

There are several cutting-type biopsy needles and the Tru-cut needle is currently the most popular. The Silverman needle, and some of its modifications, such as Murray Franklin or White, consists of a needle sheath and a double harpoon-ended stilette. The needle is inserted with the stilette within the sheath and advanced into the area to be biopsied. The harpoon-ended stilette is then advanced beyond the tip of the sheath, which causes it to flare laterally thus encompassing a small section of tissue. Thereafter, the sheath is advanced while holding the stilette steady, and the whole needle is withdrawn. The biopsy is lodged between the two leaves of the stilette.

The Tru-cut biopsy needle is a disposable, factory pre-assembled needle. It too has a needle sheath and an obturator with a bevelled tip and, immediately behind, a biopsy slot. Fully extended, the obturator is 2.8 cm long. The needle is operated by a T-shaped plastic handle and the obturator by a small mobile handle directly behind. The needle is inserted with the obturator retracted. When the tissue to the biopsied is reached, the obturator is pushed in and then while holding it steady the sheath is advanced, and the whole needle withdrawn. The specimen thus obtained is 2 cm long and approximately 1.5 mm in diameter. The success of the Tru-cut needle lies in that it is disposable and sharp, and in the good-sized, undistorted biopsy material obtained.

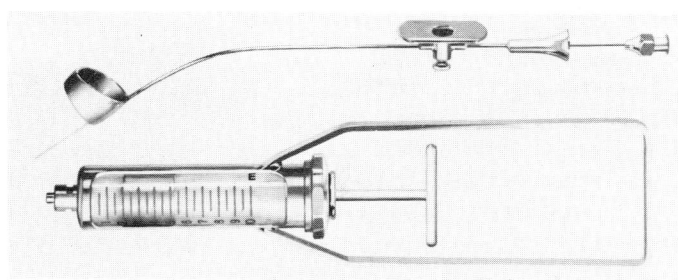

Menghini, G. (1958) One-second needle biopsy of the liver. *Gastroenterology*, **54**, 241.
Silverman, I. (1938) A new biopsy needle. *American Journal of Surgery*, **40**, 671.
Roberts, J.G., Preece, P.E., Bolton, P.M., Baum, M. and Hughes, L.E. (1975) *Clinical Oncology* **1**, 297.
Westaby, D. and Williams, R. (1980) How to biopsy the liver. *British Journal of Hospital Medicine*, May 1980, 527.

3.4 Biopsy punch forceps

Biopsy forceps remove a piece of tissue by the occlusion of two cupped jaws and are especially suitable for mucosal

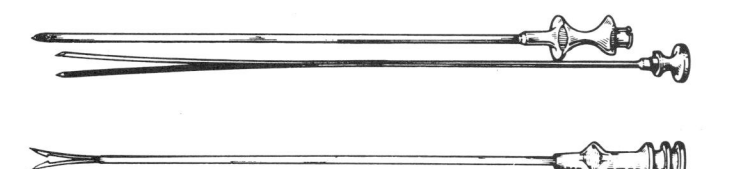

Fig.39 Franzen needle for prostatic biopsy

Fig.40 Silverman needle (Downs)

Fig.41 Murray Franklin modification of Silverman needle (Downs)

biopsies. In the closed position the sharp edges of the cup come into contact with that of the opposite cup. The action severs a piece of tissue within the hollow of cups.

The basket-jawed forceps, such as Yeoman or Chevalier–Jackson, have one smaller cup which fits exactly within the larger opposite cup. Cutting takes place by a shearing action as the smaller cup is closed within the larger. These forceps generally have a better cutting action than the cupped type. However, they are not as haemostatic as ordinary cupped forceps, where a twisting action is generally required to remove the specimen. The jaws can be straight or angled, as in Chevalier–Jackson forceps.

The jaws are opened and closed by two handles operated by the thumb and middle fingers of the right hand. The movement of one of the handles is transmitted to one jaw. Moving the fingers apart opens the jaws.

3.5 Trephine biopsy

The trepan was an early predecessor of the trephine. It consisted of a crown saw for cutting small pieces of bone, especially from the skull. The trephine is an improved version of this and consists of a crown saw in the centre of which is an adjustable sharp steel pin, which is fixed upon bone to steady the movement of operating. Although the trephine has been primarily used for biopsy of the skull it is also suitable, in a modified form, for bone biopsy.

Henry Turkel of Detroit designed a trephine needle for bone biopsy and this is still being used virtually unchanged. It consists of an outer cannula with a short bevelled trochar and an inner needle with a trephine edge and a clearing pilot. The outer cannula is introduced into the bone, its trochar removed and the trephine

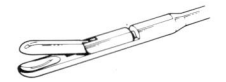

Fig.42 Lloyd Davis sigmoidoscope biopsy forceps (Downs)

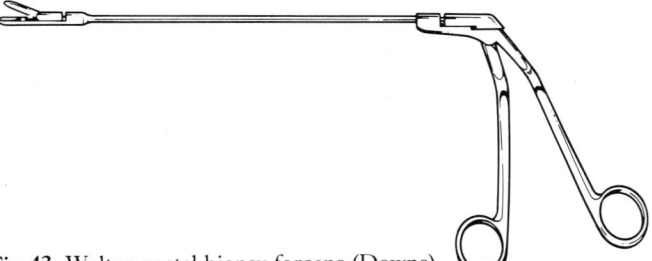

Fig.43 Walton rectal biopsy forceps (Downs)

Fig.44 Yeoman biopsy forceps (Downs)

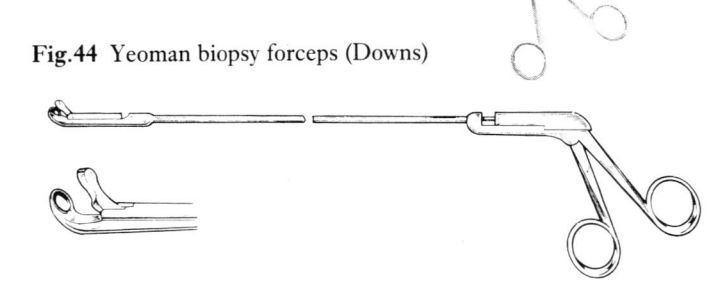

Fig.45 Chevalier–Jackson biopsy forceps (Downs)

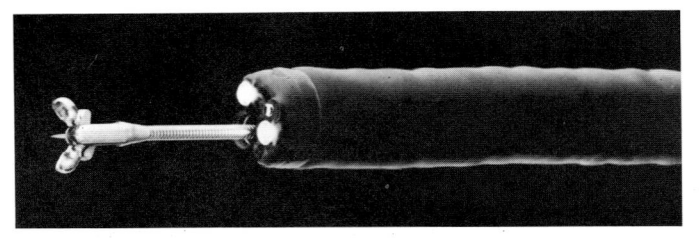

Fig.46 Distal tip of Olympus GIF-IT gastro-duodenoscope showing size of biopsy forceps (Key Med)

needle introduced. By moving the trephine needle in a circle, a cylinder of bone is carved out. This can be aspirated with a syringe if soft bone is encountered. Otherwise the bone biopsy is removed with the clearing pilot.

The Royal National Orthopaedic Hospital (RNOH) trephine is a longer instrument, used for full-thickness iliac-crest biopsy. It is distinguished by having two handles, one for steadying the outer cannula and the other for imparting circular motion to the trephine.

High-speed drill biopsy is also a form of trephine biopsy.

Fig.47 Turkel trephine (Downs)

Fig.48 R.N.O.H. trephine (Downs)

3.6 High-speed drill biopsy

This is a trephine biopsy where the trephine needle, driven by a pneumatic drill, rotates at around 15 000 revolutions per minute.

The technique is used almost exclusively for lung biopsy but may be used for other tissues. It provides a core of tissue 2.1 mm in diameter and up to 5 cm long. For obvious reasons it is preferable to open biopsy of superficial lung lesions.

The needle, with a trochar, is inserted percutaneously and when the pleura is pierced the drill is attached to the trephine. While rotating, the needle is advanced to a depth of 4–5 cms. The drill is disconnected, the syringe is attached to the needle and, while maintaining suction, the needle is withdrawn.

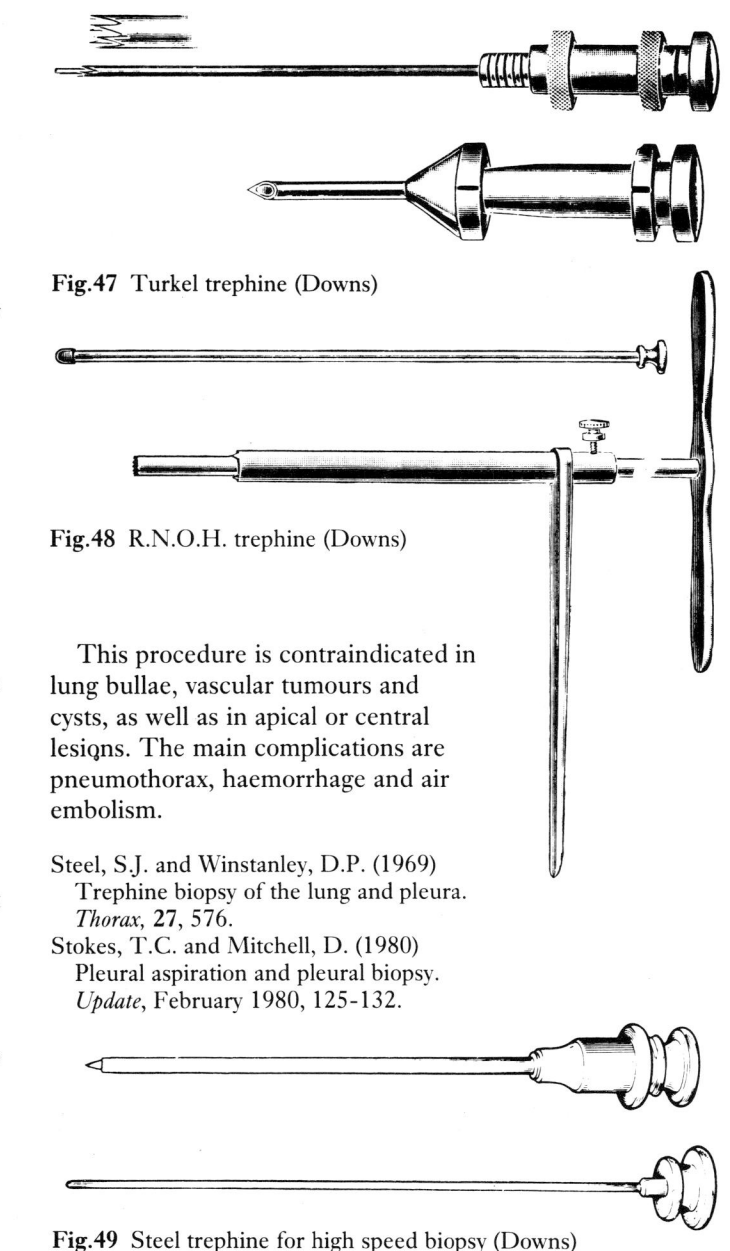

This procedure is contraindicated in lung bullae, vascular tumours and cysts, as well as in apical or central lesions. The main complications are pneumothorax, haemorrhage and air embolism.

Steel, S.J. and Winstanley, D.P. (1969) Trephine biopsy of the lung and pleura. *Thorax*, **27**, 576.
Stokes, T.C. and Mitchell, D. (1980) Pleural aspiration and pleural biopsy. *Update*, February 1980, 125-132.

Fig.49 Steel trephine for high speed biopsy (Downs)

3.7 Diathermy snare and loop

A diathermy current can be used in some cases for obtaining a biopsy. The cutting current is used in the urinary bladder to obtain biopsies of tumours. This has the advantage of complete excision of tumour down to muscle, thus providing a suitable specimen for histological staging. At the same time, cutting diathermy has a haemostatic effect which can be supplemented by a coagulating current.

Gastrointestinal polypoid tumours can be removed endoscopically with the snare loop diathermy. This consists of wire loop contained within an insulating sheath. The loop is passed over the polyp and then tightened over its stalk. While tightening the loop and gently exerting traction, a coagulating current is applied. This coagulates any vessels and slowly cuts through the stalk.

The absolute contraindication for this procedure is large polyps in the colon and flat lesions. Diathermy must not be used within the bowel prepared with Mannitol as there have been reports of explosions due to methane ignition.

3.8 Crosby–Kugler intestinal biopsy

In 1957 Crosby and Kugler described a suction biopsy capsule for biopsy of the small intestine.

The capsule has one or two biopsy holes. Within the capsule is a spring-loaded piston blade which is fired by suction. Suction applied by a syringe first sucks in a piece of mucosa, which is then cut off by the activated piston blade.

The capsule is swallowed by mouth and when 60 cm of the tubing has been passed the patient is positioned on his right side while encouraged to swallow another 20 cm of tubing. Further passage of the capsule is performed under fluoroscopic control. If passage through the duodenum is difficult, an internal stiffening wire may be of help.

After the capsule has passed through the duodenum the patient is positioned on his left side, and when the capsule is seen to be in the jejunum it is 'fired'.

Crosby, W.H. and Kugler, H.W. (1957) *American Journal of Digestive Diseases*, **2**, 236.

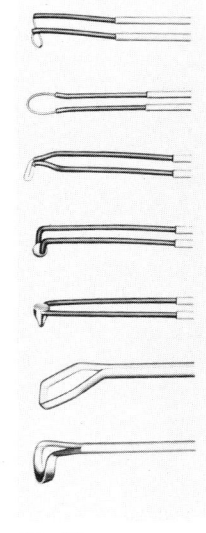

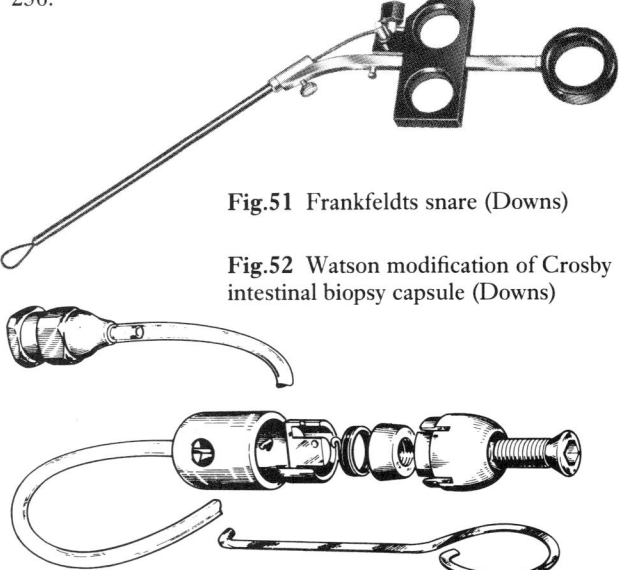

Fig.50 Resectoscope loops (Storz)

Fig.51 Frankfeldts snare (Downs)

Fig.52 Watson modification of Crosby intestinal biopsy capsule (Downs)

3.9 Cryobiopsy

The advantages of taking biopsies of superficial lesions using this technique are many. The procedure can be carried out in out-patient departments and does not require anaesthesia.

Because of the haemostatic effect of freezing, diathermy, or any other form of haemostasis, is not required. The biopsy can then be formally excised or biopsied with puch forceps or a biopsy needle.

Friable tissues are less likely to be damaged and in small lesions the cryoprobe itself has a therapeutic effect in destroying pathological tissue.

Part 2   Therapeutic Instruments

Chapter 4 Vascular Access

4.1 Tourniquet
4.2 Vascular cannulae and catheters
4.3 Embolectomy catheters
4.4 Percutaneous transluminal angioplasty
4.5 Therapeutic embolisation
4.6 Caval filters
4.7 Pulmonary artery flotation catheters
4.8 External arteriovenous shunts
4.9 Intra-aortic balloon pump

4.1 Tourniquet

The simple tourniquet, an elastic band, is in daily use in all hospitals. It is used for venepuncture or insertion of peripheral venous cannulae. The tourniquet was, however, originally developed to control haemorrhage.

Over the centuries bleeding from open wounds was initially controlled by local pressure and bandage, and gradually this technique was replaced by boiling oil or cauterising iron. Paré used a ligature for the first time $c.1640$. In 1674 Morell used a field garotte to stop haemorrhage. This was a simple cord with a wooden rod used to twist the cord to tighten it. From the end of the seventeenth century the garotte was used in amputation.

In 1718 Jean Louis Petit developed a screw compressor which exerted pressure over the vessel, and he named this instrument a tourniquet. The pressure could be varied and there was no need for assistance. From there on, many different designs were developed but most of them eventually consisted of a strong linen or leather strap with a metal compressor consisting of a cog-and-wheel mechanism.

Modern tourniquets are not much different from their antique predecessors. The Samway anchor pattern tourniquet consists of a length of rubber tubing and a T-shaped metal piece around which the tubing is fastened. Another commonly used tourniquet is the 'quick release' type. The strap can be tightened over a metal buckle, and a spring-loaded hinge allows instant release of tension.

These tourniquets have two major disadvantages: the pressure exerted is very localised and is inaccurate. These problems can be avoided by the use of the inflatable cuff tourniquet; this exerts pressure over a wide area, thus

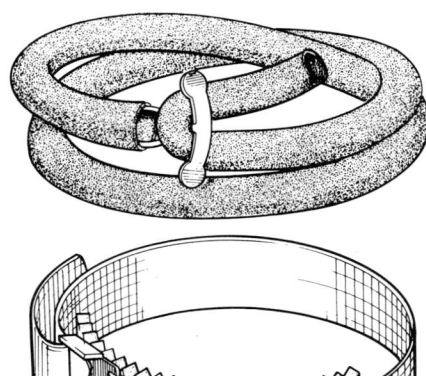

Fig.53 Samway anchor tourniquet (Downs)

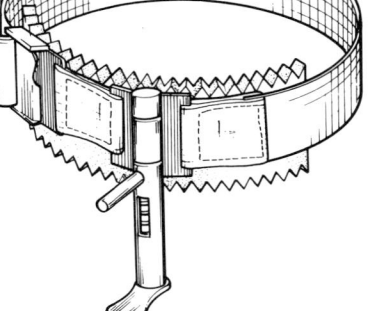

Fig.54 Qualter 'quick release' tourniquet (Downs)

avoiding damage to skin and vessels, and pressure within can be monitored and altered at will.

Tourniquets are used mainly in limb surgery rather than in emergency, where complete exsanguination is required for prolonged periods of time. Tourniquets should be used with care. Inadequate pressure may result in venous congestion, oedema and even Volkmann's contracture. When applied properly, occlusion of circulation should be used for limited periods of time, with regular release and reinflation to prevent irreversible ischaemia. The total time of occulsion (tourniquet time) must always be recorded. At the end of an operation the tourniquet must be removed rather than just loosened. Many cases are recorded when a tourniquet was discovered *in situ* hours after surgery had been completed, resulting not only in the loss of a limb but also in loss of life due to the crush syndrome. In such cases it is imperative that the tourniquet is left *in situ* and removed after amputation of the limb distal to the tourniquet.

4.2 Vascular cannulae and catheters

One of the most important therapeutic advances in medicine and surgery was the introduction of plastic cannulae and catheters, enabling safe access to venous and arterial circulation for a variety of purposes. Without these, modern therapeutic medicine would be unthinkable. Yet just over a decade ago, cutdown was commonplace and routine percutaneous venous catheterisation unthinkable. Venous cannulae were all metal, resterilisable and clumsy.

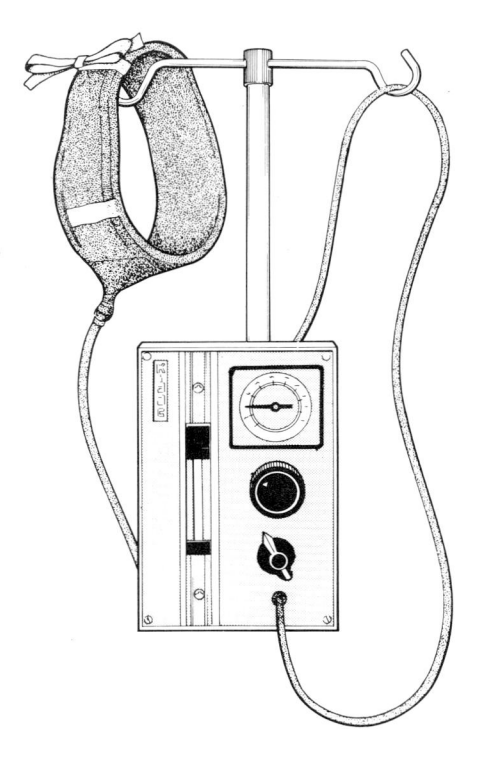

Fig.55 Kidde standard pneumatic tourniquet (Downs)

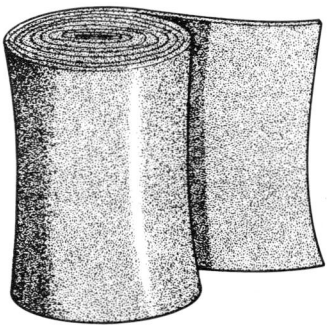

Fig.56 Esmarch bandage (Downs)

The current choice of vascular cannulae and catheters is vast and bears witness to the ingenuity of the medical technological revolution.

Vascular catheters and cannulae can be broadly divided into peripheral and central. Peripheral cannulae are short plastic sheaths splinted by a central hollow metal needle. The proximal end of the cannula usually has a device for syringe or tubing attachment and may have a separate inlet, with or without a filter, for infusion of drugs or for flushing. This cannula is suitable for cannulation of superficial arteries and veins. The materials used in the manufacture of cannulae are PVC, polyethylene, tetrafluoroethylene or fluoroethylene propylene. There has been a swing towards using fluorethylene propylene (Teflon) because this material causes less venous reaction than others. In some cases the cannula is a metal needle (Butterfly) with a plastic end and plastic tubing, and its use is almost entirely limited to short-term infusion of drugs, as in anaesthesia.

By convention, the cannula sizes are identified in gauge (G) numbers and are colour coded. Rather confusingly, increasing gauge numbers signify smaller diameter; thus 12G has an external diameter of 2.6 mm, 16G of 1.6 mm and 22G of 0.71 mm.

Central venous catheterisation is a technique of catheter placement into the superior vena cava, right atrium or inferior vena cava. The large veins of the body, especially the superior vena cava, are suitable for monitoring of central venous pressure, convenient and frequent blood sampling, rapid infusion of fluids in an emergency, and infusion of hyperosmolar fluids.

The basic equipment consists of a needle with or without cannula, and a catheter. The catheter is a long, flexible tube and can be inserted through or over the needle, through a cannula or over guidewires.

The best known catheter-through-needle is the drum cartridge catheter. The needle is inserted into a vein and the catheter, wound on a drum, is advanced into the vessel via the needle lumen. One disadvantage of this technique is that the catheter is smaller than the needle and subsequently there may be leakage of blood around the puncture site. The main drawback, however, is the possiblity of the catheter being sheared off if an attempt to withdraw it is made.

The catheter-over-needle device was developed to avoid the risk of catheter shearing. Effectively it is a long cannula. The needle lies within the catheter and both are inserted into a vein. Once in the lumen the needle is then withdrawn and the catheter advanced further. The length of the catheter is limited and, since the needle protrudes beyond its tip, a flashback of blood may not necessarily indicate that the catheter is within the vessel lumen. Because the catheter has to be moderately rigid, injury to the vein can take place. Leakage of blood around the puncture site is uncommon because the needle is smaller than the catheter.

THERAPEUTIC INSTRUMENTS

The catheter-through-cannula device has some advantages over the previously mentioned devices. Venepuncture is carried out with a cannula and needle. Aspiration with a syringe ascertains the position within the lumen, the needle is removed and the catheter advanced into the vein through the cannula. The main disadvantages of this technique are the possibility that the cannula tip may not be within the lumen and that since the catheter size is smaller than that of the cannula there may be blood leakage around the puncture site.

The catheter-over-guidewire device was introduced by Seldinger for percutaneous arteriography in 1953. The flexible guidewire is inserted through a needle and the needle is removed. The catheter is inserted into the vein over the guidewire. Larger catheters such as Swan–Ganz can be introduced with the help of a tapered vein dilator. The advantage of this technique is that a smaller needle is required for the initial vein puncture and that since the catheter is larger than the guidewire, leakage around the puncture site is negligible. However, this device is more complex and expensive.

With the wider use of long-term parenteral nutrition, central venous catheters have been developed specifically for this purpose. These catheters are generally larger in diameter and are designed to minimise infection spreading along the catheter. The Broviac catheter is a silastic catheter with a Dacron cuff which is

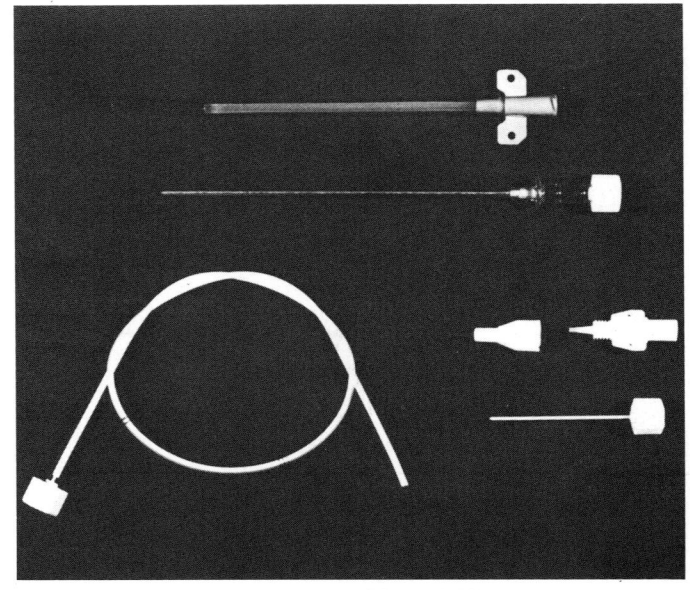

Fig.57 Catheter-through-cannula (Vygon UK)

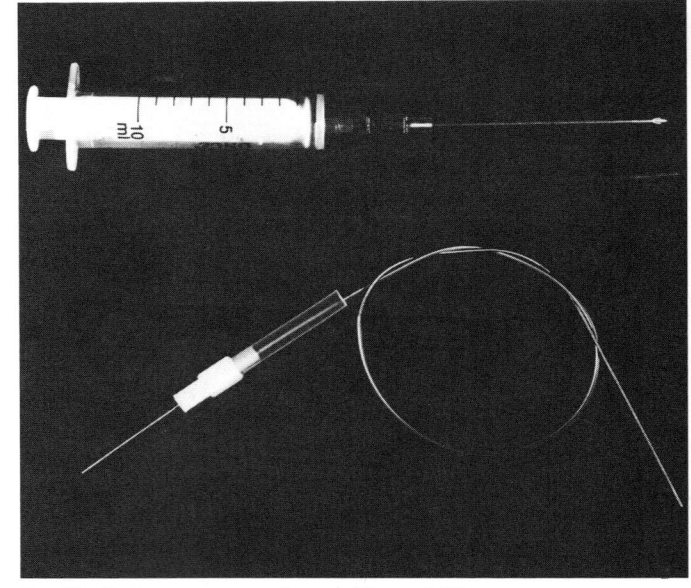

Fig.58 Catheter-over-guidewire (Vygon UK)

buried subcutaneously. Fibrosis around the cuff prevents external infection from spreading along the periphery of the catheter.

The Hickman catheter is a modification of the Broviac catheter and was designed specifically for venous access in marrow transplant recipients. It has a larger internal diameter, thus allowing easy infusion as well as withdrawal of blood, and is less likely to clot up. Although it is frequently inserted via a cutdown into the cephalic vein it can be inserted percutaneously using the catheter-over-guidewire technique with a vein dilator.

Most modern catheters are made of silastic because of its softness and lack of thrombogenicity. For that reason silastic is preferable to Teflon, polyester-based polymers or polypropylene.

Willatts, S. (1980) How to cannulate a peripheral artery. *British Journal of Hospital Medicine*, 1980, 628-630.

Smith, B.L. (1978) Intravenous techniques *British Journal of Hospital Medicine*, 1978, 454, 458.

Jones, D.F. (1979) Central venous catheterisation. *Hospital Update*, 1979, 485-496

Rosen, M., Latto, I.P. and Ng, W.S. (1981) *Handbook of Percutaneous Central Venous Catheterisation*. W.B. Saunders, Philadelphia.

Broviac, J.W. Cole, J.J. and Schribner, B.H. (1973) A silicone rubber atrial catheter for prolonged parenteral alimentation. *Surgery, Gynecology & Obstetrics*, **136**, 602-606

Jackson, M.A. (1983) Long-term parenteral nutrition. *British Journal of Hospital Medicine*, 1983, 105-116.

Hickman, R.O., Buckman, C.D. and Clift, R.A. (1979) A modified right atrial catheter for access to the venous system in marrow transplant recipients. *Surgery, Gynecology & Obstetrics*, **148**, 871-875.

Seldinger, S.I. (1953) Catheter replacement of needle in percutaneous arteriography: a new technique. *Acta Radiologica*, **39**, 368.

4.3 Embolectomy catheters

The current successful treatment of peripheral arterial embolism is entirely due to a simple and brilliant device first described in 1963 — the Fogarty balloon catheter.

The first successful femoral embolectomy was described in 1936 by Labey. Prior to the introduction of the Fogarty catheter, arterial embolectomy was a largely unsuccessful procedure, with poor results and high mortality. Numerous methods and devices had been used. Keeley and Rooney used retrograde milking by means of rubber bandages applied tightly to the limb. Shaw described a corkscrew-type of wire for extraction of emboli and others used adapted vein strippers. Retrograde flushing was described by Lerman. Yet the introduction of a thin, flexible catheter with a small inflatable balloon at the distal end altered the prognosis of this disease and revolutionised vascular surgery.

The Fogarty catheter is a semirigid plastic tube of 3–7 Ch size and usually 80 cm long, although other lengths are available. The tip is blunt and several millimetres proximal to it is an inflatable balloon with a capacity of 0.2 to 2.5 ml. A metal stylet is contained within the lumen and serves to stiffen the catheter during its storage and insertion. After removal of the stylet a syringe is attached to the Luer fitting at the proximal end of the catheter; this serves to inflate or deflate the balloon.

The most important points to remember while using the catheter are never to use force while trying to pass it and never to over-inflate the balloon. Failure to observe these principles can result in severe damage to the vessel.

The technique itself is simple. The operation is usually performed under local anaesthetic. The vessel is exposed and a longitudinal or transverse arteriotomy carried out. Prior to passing the catheter of suitable size it is essential to inflate the balloon to ensure that it is intact and to determine its optimal size. The catheter should be passed by the surgeon himself, whether proximally or distally, the balloon inflated and catheter withdrawn slowly. Should resistance increase as the catheter is being withdrawn the balloon may have to be deflated to prevent vessel damage. As mentioned previously, the main complication is vascular damage due to overinflation of the balloon or the use of excessive force during the passage of the catheter.

Lerman, J., Miller, F.R. and Lund, C.C. (1939) Arterial embolism and embolectomy. *Journal of the American Medical Association*, **94**, 1128

Keeley, J.L. and Rooney, J.A. (1951) Retrograde milking — an adjunct in technique of embolectomy. *Annals of Surgery*, **184**, 1022

Fogarty, T.J., Cranley, J.J., Krause, R.J., Strasser, E.S. and Hafner, C.D. (1963) *Surgery, Gynecology & Obstetrics*, CXVi, 241

Fogarty, T.J. and Cranley, J.J. (1965) Catheter technique for arterial embolectomy. *Annals of Surgery*, **161**, 325

4.4 Percutaneous transluminal angioplasty

The first attempt to dilate an arterial stenosis was made in 1964 by Dotter and Judkins, who used coaxial catheters, where a larger catheter was passed over a smaller one to produce the desired effect. Attempts to use Fogarty catheters were largely unsuccessful due to the balloon's elasticity. In 1974 Grüntzig and Hopff introduced a new flexible catheter with a non-elastic PVC balloon.

Since then the technique of transluminal percutaneous angioplasty has become established as an alternative to current surgical techniques for the management of arterial strictures and stenoses.

The catheter is flexible, with a double lumen to allow the insertion of a central guidewire and independent inflation of the balloon. The balloon is made of polyvinylchloride or more recently from stronger polyethylene, resulting in relative inelasticity under high pressure of inflation. It can be safely inflated up to 400 kPa.

Catheters are supplied in different lengths and diameters with balloons of varying length and diameter. The guide wires are also supplied in various shapes to allow cannulation of stenoses at distant sites.

The procedure is carried out under local anaesthesia, fluoroscopic control and heparin anticoagulation. The stenosed segment of an artery is approached in a retrograde or antigrade manner and after cannulation of the access artery the guide wire is passed through the stricture.

The Güntzig catheter is passed over the wire and the two radiopaque markers are positioned so that each lies on either side of stenosed segment. The balloon is inflated several times with a dilute contrast medium. The medium must be completely evacuated before removal of the catheter.

Percutaneous transluminal angioplasty is now firmly established in peripheral vascular disease, and coronary and renal artery disease. Its mortality is comparable to equivalent surgical procedure and morbidity is lower. Complications are rarely serious, although complete rupture of the dilated segment does occur. The main complications are related to the puncture site, haematoma and haemorrhage being the commonest. Rarely, peripheral embolism, arterial thrombosis, subintimal dissection and false aneurysm at the puncture site occur. It must be stressed that this procedure is suitable for a small percentage of patients with arterial disease. Although patency following angioplasty is not as good as that following traditional surgery, such as femoro-popliteal bypass, it would not be suprising if this state of affairs became reversed over the next decade.

Dotter, C.T. and Judkins, M.P. (1964) Transluminal treatment of arteriosclerotic obstruction.
Kumpe, D. and Grüntzig, A. (1979) Technique of percutaneous transluminal angioplasty with Grüntzig balloon catheter. *American Journal of Roentgerology, Radium Therapy and Nuclear Medicine*, **124**, 428-435.
Dacie, J.E. (1981) Percutaneous transluminal angioplasty. *British Journal of Hospital Medicine*, 1981, 314-324
Zeitler, E., Grüntzig, A. and Schoop, W. (eds) (1978) *Percutaneous Vascular Recanalisation*. Springer-Verlag, Berlin.

4.5 Therapeutic embolisation

Therapeutic embolisation is a technique of deliberate occlusion of blood vessels by materials introduced via a selectively placed catheter.

With increasing complexity of vascular catheters and skill of radiologists to introduce them into the most inaccessible vessels it became obvious that artificial embolisation would become an important therapeutic technique.

The catheters used are the same as for selective angiography and are introduced percutaneously using the Seldinger technique. Prior to embolisation, angiography is essential to display the anatomy of the blood supply. The catheter should be sited as accurately as possible to avoid damage to adjacent structures. The technique itself is simple. Having ascertained the position of the catheter by fluoroscopy, embolic material is injected via the lumen of the catheter into the vessel, under fluoroscopic control. Should the material used be non-opaque it must be injected with a contrast medium. To avoid inadvertent embolisation of other structures, special balloon catheters are used. Catheterisation of vessels which is difficult with the standard catheter guidance system can be achieved by 'floating' a small balloon catheter into these vessels.

The materials used for embolisation range from autologous materials, such as smooth muscle, blood clot and fat, to artificial materials such as steel balls, beads, gelatin sponges, instantly setting polymers, etc.. The ideal substance should be radiopaque and injectable, sterile and non-toxic, thrombogenic and stable. None of the above materials fulfils these criteria and some may be hazardous to use. The instantly setting polymers, for example, may set so quickly that the tip of the catheter may be incorporated in the embolus. Therapeutic embolisation is indicated in haemorrhage, tumours, either palliative or pre-operative embolisation, vascular malformations and aneurysms.

The main complications are pain and low-grade fever. Infection and retrograde propagation of thrombosis are uncommon but should always be kept in mind during the post-operative period.

Dick, R. (1977) Radiology now: therapeutic angiographic embolisation. *British Journal of Radiology*, **50**, 241-242.

Allison, D.J. (1978) Therapeutic embolisation. *British Journal of Hospital Medicine*, **20**, 707-715.

Gianturco, C., Anderson, J.H. and Wallace, S. (1975) Mechanical devices for arterial occlusion. *American Journal of Roentgenology, Radium Therapy and Nuclear Medicine*, **124**, 428-435.

Allison, D.J. (1980) Therapeutic embolisation and venous sampling. *Recent Advances in Surgery*, **10**, 27-64.

4.6 Caval filters

Recurrent pulmonary embolism in patients with deep vein thrombosis, in spite of adequate anticoagulation, presents a major therapeutic problem.

Ochsner and DeBakey popularised surgical ligation of the inferior vena cava for this condition in the early 1940s and this technique has been widely practised until very recently. This operation has, however, many disadvantages. Acute ligation of the inferior vena cava can halve the cardiac output and formation of collateral venous channels around the ligated segment provides not only a collateral pathway for blood but also further emboli. The ligation itself causes significant stasis, which may potentiate thrombosis and embolism in a proportion of patients.

Attempts to maintain patency of the cava while providing protection from embolism led to the introduction of caval plication and filtration. Although these operations overcame some of the problems of caval ligation, such major surgical procedures in the severely ill and anticoagulated patients carried a very high mortality.

In 1967 Mobin-Uddin introduced a transvenous method of placing an umbrella filter into the inferior vena cava, which immediately replaced the previous surgical operations. This filter was, however, associated with a high incidence of caval thrombosis, stasis, collateralisation and recurrent embolism. In 1973 Greenfield introduced a new filter which was specifically designed to maintain caval patency while providing protection from embolism. This too can be introduced via the jugular vein as well as the femoral vein.

The technique of insertion is similar for both filters. Under local or general anaesthesia the internal jugular vein is exposed in the neck and venotomy is carried out. A guide wire is passed through the venotomy and positioned in the inferior vena cava. The rigid end of the guide wire is then passed retrogradely through the

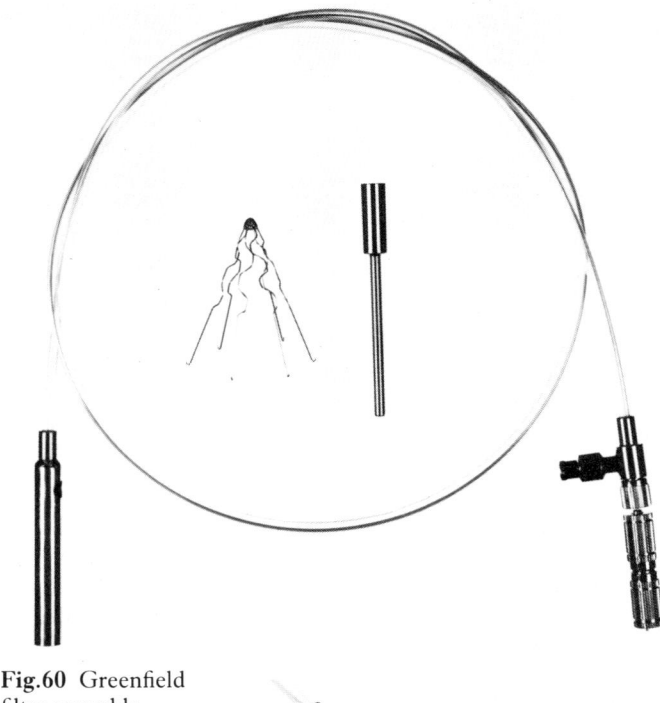

Fig.60 Greenfield filter assembly

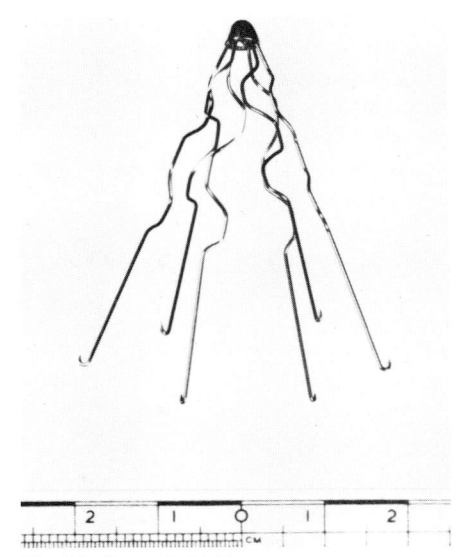

Fig.59 Greenfield filter

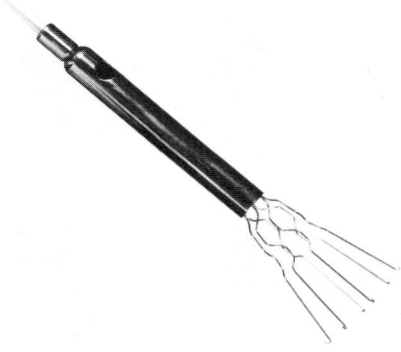

Fig.61 Greenfield filter

catheter−carrier assembly. The inserter is passed over the guide wire to the vena cava and the filter is fired by holding the stylet and withdrawing the catheter. Both the guide wire and the catheter are removed and the venotomy repaired.

The main complications are misplacement and migration, the latter being less likely with the Greenfield filter. Filter penetration of the caval wall may occur but is rare.

Ochsner, A. & DeBakey M. (1943) Intravenous clotting and its sequelae. *Surgery*, **14**, 679.

Cimochowski, G.E., Evans, R.H., Zarins, K.C., Chien-Tai, Lu and Demeester, T.R. (1980) Greenfield filter versus Mobin-Uddin umbrella. *Journal of Thoracic and Cardiovascular Surgery*, **79**, 358-365.

Mobin-Uddin, K., McLean, R. and Jude, J.R. (1969) A new catheter technique of interruption of inferior vena cava for prevention of pulmonary embolism. *Annals of Surgery*, **35**, 889.

Scurr, J.H., Jarrett, P.E.M. and Wastell, C. (1983) The treatment of recurrent pulmonary embolism: experience with the Kimray Greenfield vena cava filter. *Annals of the Royal College of Surgeons of England*, **65**, 233-234.

Greenfield, L.J., Steward, J.R. and Crute, S. (1983) Improved technique for insertion of Greenfield vena cava filter. *Surgery, Gynecology & Obstetrics*, **156**, 217-219.

4.7 Pulmonary artery flotation catheters

Severely ill patients with complex cardiac problems may require cardiac monitoring in the form of pressure measurements because of disparity between the right and left sides of the heart.

It is well known that central venous pressure, in the presence of normal tricuspid valve, equals the right ventricular end — diastolic pressure. Equally, the pulmonary artery wedge pressure relates closely to the left ventricular end — diastolic pressure. These pressures can be used as an index of the right and left ventricular function.

Catheterisation of the right heart was first performed by Forssmann in 1929. A true bedside pulmonary artery catheterisation became possible in 1970 when Swan and Ganz introduced a flow-directible catheter with an inflatable balloon. The catheter, 5−7 FG in size, is 80−110 cm long. There are markings on the catheter to indicate the distance from the tip. The catheter is inserted via any major vein, usually the subclavian, using the cutdown or Seldinger technique. The catheter is advanced into the superior vena cava and attached to a pressure transducer. The balloon is inflated and, while introducing the catheter further, is carried with the blood flow into and through the right heart. As soon as pressure recordings resemble those of pulmonary artery wedge pressure, with the balloon inflated, the position of the catheter is checked with a chest X-ray or fluoroscopy. The guide wire is removed and the catheter secured.

The main complications of this

technique are infection, pulmonary embolism and infarction, and knotting of the catheter. Embolism occurs when the catheter is neglected. Large clots form and these are dislodged in an attempt to flush the catheter with heparinised solution.

Pulmonary infarction is the result of pulmonary artery occlusion by the balloon or spontaneous wedging of the catheter. Knotting the catheter is usually associated with catheterisation of dilated right heart and should be prevented by observing the absence of pressure waves beyond 30 cm of insertion.

Swan, H.J.C., Ganz, W., Forrester, T., Marcus, H., Diamond, G. and Chouette, D. (1970) *New England Journal of Medicine*, **283**, 447.

George, R.J.D. (1980) How to insert a flotation catheter. *British Journal of Hospital Medicine*, **123**, 296.

George, R.J.D. and Banks, R.A. (1983) Bedside measurements of pulmonary capillary wedge pressure. *British Journal of Hospital Medicine*, March 1983, 286.

4.8 External arteriovenous shunts

The haemodialysis machine was first used clinically in 1955, by Kolff. Access to circulation at that time required cutdown on artery and vein and this precluded the use of dialysis for chronic renal failure. In 1960, Scribner, Dillard and Quinton described the first external A−V shunt made of Teflon−silastic. This device was replaced by the Brescia−Cimino subcutaneous A−V fistula because the external fistula was unsuitable for use in chronic intermittent dialysis.

The external A−V shunt consists of arterial and venous cannulae connected by shunt tubing. The arterial and venous tips must be of appropriate size to prevent leakage of blood or vessel damage. The tips must also be sufficiently large to provide adequate flow into and out of the dialysis machine and the arterial diameter must be smaller than the venous end, otherwise ultrafiltration and bleeding into dialysis will take place.

The Quinton−Dillard−Scribner shunt consists of silastic tubing with tips made of Teflon. The ends are placed end-to-side into the vessels and subcutaneous rings serve to prevent rotation of the tubing during use. In an attempt to prolong the longevity of external A−V shunts, a number of improved shunts are in use.

The Allen−Brown A−V shunt has a Dacron sleeve and Dacron knitted prosthesis. The Dacron prosthesis is sewn on the vessel end-to-end or end-to-side and needs to be pre-clotted prior to insertion.

The Buselmeier shunt is shorter and has a fixed U-shape which makes it suitable only for radial and cephalic and posterior tibial and saphenous vessels. It is said to have higher flow rate than other shunts.

The Thomas shunt was designed for larger vessels, namely the femoral artery and vein. It is very similar to the Allen−Brown shunt in that it employs a knitted Dacron end and requires formal vascular anastomosis.

External A−V shunts are used mainly in acute haemodialysis, i.e. acute renal failure, as well as in patients on home dialysis who are unable to introduce needles into internal shunts. The main complications of these shunts are clotting, infection and bleeding.

Graham, W.B. (1977) Historical aspects of haemodialysis. *Transplant Proceedings*, **9**,
Kolff W.J. (1965) The first clinical experience with the artificial kidney. *Annals of Internal Medicine*, **62**, 608.
Quinton, W.E., Dillard, D.H. and Scribner, B.H. (1960) Cannulation of blood vessels for prolonged haemodialysis. *Transactions of the American Society for Artificial Internal Organs*, **6**, 104.
Brescia, M.J., Cimino, J.E., Appel, K. and Hummich, B.J. (1966) Chronic haemodialysis using venepuncture and a surgically created arteriovenous fistula. *New England Journal of Medicine*, **275** (20), 1089.
Ozeran, R.S. (1983) Construction and care of external arteriovenous shunts. In: *Vascular Access Surgery* (ed. Wilson, S.E. and Owens, M.L.). Yearbook Medical, Chicago.
Reilly, D.T. and Wood, R.F.M. (1982) Arteriovenous fistulae for haemodialysis. *Hospital Update*, 1982, 693-706.

4.9 Intra-aortic balloon pump

Intra-aortic balloon pumps have been used since the early 1970s for temporary circulatory support of patients with cardiogenic shock following myocardial infarction or open-heart surgery, or, prophylactically, before emergency surgery or open-heart surgery in patients with severe coronary artery disease.

The intra-aortic pump is inserted into the thoracic aorta via a femoral artery either through a cutdown or percutaneously. The balloon is inflated, with helium or carbon dioxide, and deflated by a pump synchronised with the patient's ECG or arterial pressure recording. Inflation takes place during diastole and deflation during systole.

The result is an elevated aortic pressure in diastole, thus increasing the coronary blood flow, and depressed aortic pressure during systole, leading to decreased left ventricular load and myocardial oxygen consumption.

The closer the balloon is to the aortic valve, the greater is the elevation in the mean aortic diastolic pressures. As expected, the size of the balloon has significant effects on the change in diastolic pressures. However, large balloons carry the risk of trauma to the aortic wall and damage to erythrocytes. In order to prevent too high a lateral pressure during inflation, dual or triple-chamber balloons have been introduced.

Balooki, H. (ed) (1977) *Clinical Applications of the Intra-aortic Balloon Pump*. Futura Press, New York.
Tobias, M.A. (1981) Intra-aortic balloon pumps. *British Journal of Hospital Medicine*, 1981, 542-548.

Chapter 5 Drains and Splints

5.1 Gastric and intestinal tubes
5.2 Oesophageal tubes
5.3 Abdominal drains
5.4 Chest drains
5.5 Urological catheters
5.6 Peritoneal dialysis catheters
5.7 Peritoneo-venous shunt
5.8 Biliary drains
5.9 Tracheostomy and endotracheal tubes

5.1 Gastric and intestinal tubes

Tubes may have to be passed into the stomach, or even beyond, for decompression, sampling or delivery of drugs or food. The least sophisticated is the gastric lavage tube, so often used in casualty departments for stomach washouts. It is a wide-bore rubber tube with a suitably round tip at one end and a funnel attached at the other.

Ryle's gastroduodenal tube is most commonly used for decompression of the stomach following abdominal surgery or for obstruction. It differs from Rehfuss's tube in that the tube is moulded in one piece with a small steel ball weight concealed in its tip. Rehfuss's tube has a detachable metal suction end. Modern Ryle's tubes are transparent and made of Portex.

The Miller–Abbott tube was designed for decompression or sampling of the proximal small intestine. It is about 3 m long and has an inflatable balloon at the tip. It is passed under fluoroscopic control, with the patient being tipped and turned during the process. It is very rarely used now.

Nasogastric tubes are uncomfortable and distressing, and may damage the lower oesophagus. Their long-term use is undesirable. Recently, fine silastic nasogastric tubes have been introduced specifically for enteral feeding. These fine-bore tubes are inserted with a flexible wire introducer, which is removed when the catheter is *in situ*. The position of the tip is ascertained either by testing the aspirate for acid or radiologically. The tube is comfortable and can be left unchanged for many weeks.

5.2 Oesophageal tubes

There are two types of oesophageal tubes: prosthetic and compression. Prosthetic tubes are designed to splint a stricture, almost invariably malignant. One of the first oesophageal tubes was introduced by Charles Symonds in 1885 and was made of solid gum elastic. Its upper end was funnel shaped to maintain the tube in position above the obstruction. A silk thread was left attached to it so that the tube could easily be removed and cleaned. The main disadvantage of this tube was its stiffness, making it uncomfortable, and it also became dislodged easily. The first self-retaining tube was described by Guisez in 1914. It was made of rubber and its distal end resembled that of the de Pezzer catheter, which was stretched over an introducer and passed through a rigid oesophagoscope.

In 1924 Souttar described a tube which was made of coiled German silver. This tube was flexible, self-retaining and light. However, it was narrow and had a tendency to displace itself distally. It is still used and may be introduced via a rigid oesophagoscope using a special ring retainer and introducer.

From the 1950s until quite recently, the most popular oesophageal tube was that of Mousseau, which was passed blindly through the mouth attached to a nasogastric tube and pulled down into position through a formal gastrotomy. When in position its distal end was trimmed to a suitable length and sutured to the gastric fundus.

Recent techniques of oesophageal tube insertion are based on the use of a guide wire inserted through the stricture under direct vision. This technique reduces the risk of perforation and false passage. The Nottingham introducer is designed to pass over the Puestow guide wire. It consists of an inner flexible stainless steel tube with an expanding Delrin plastic cup attached behind a flexible spring tip.

A second spiral tube, with an expanded olivary end, is inserted over this tube. The second tube expands the Delrin cup and retains the distal end of the prosthetic tube. The procedure is carried out under sedation or general anaesthesia. A guide wire is passed through the stricture and is subsequently dilated using the Eder–Puestow technique. The guide wire is removed and the stricture endoscopically examined to assess its length. The guide wire is reinserted. A tube of suitable length is selected and mounted on the Nottingham introducer. The funnel is engaged with a rammer. After adequate lubrication the assembled introducer and tube are inserted over

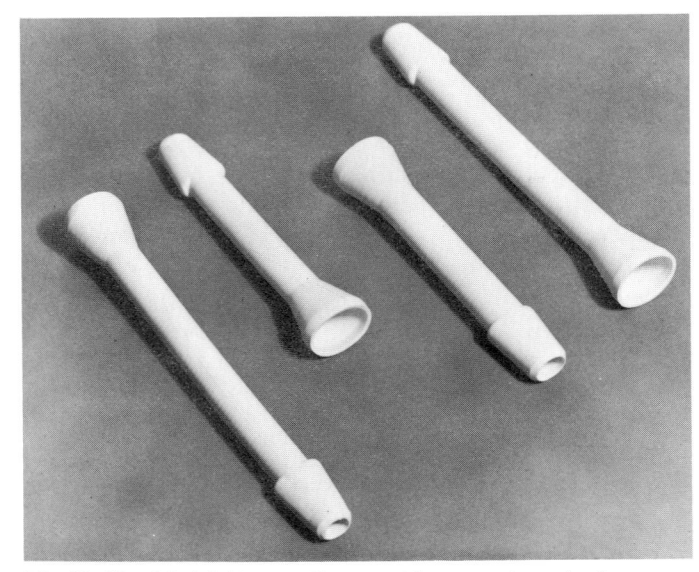

Fig.62 Key Med Atkinson silicone rubber oesophageal tubes

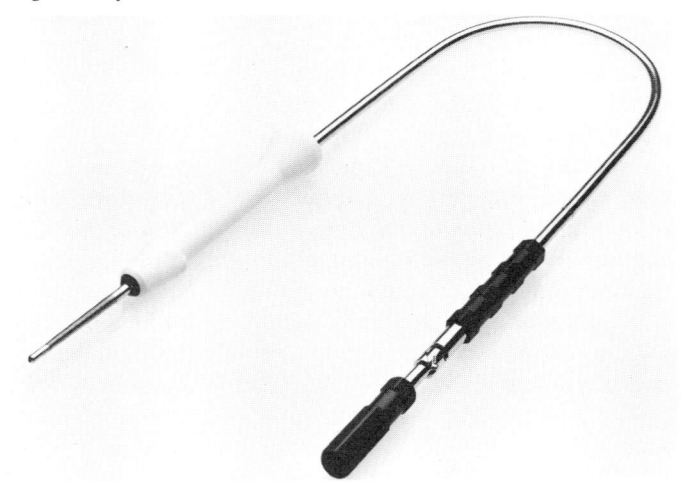

Fig.63 An Atkinson oesophageal tube mounted on the Nottingham introducer (Key Med)

the guide wire for a selected distance; the introducer is released from the tube and removed together with the guide wire, holding the tube in position with the rammer. The rammer is then disengaged from the tube's funnel and removed. The position of the tube is checked endoscopically or radiologically.

Modern prosthetic tubes are made of plastic or latex rubber for minimal irritation. They are radiopaque to enable their position to be checked. The lumen should be at least 1 cm in diameter. The proximal end is funnel-shaped to prevent distal displacement and most tubes have a distal retaining device too. The Atkinson tube, for example, designed for endoscopic insertion, has a conical distal projection.

Although it is possible to control bleeding from oesophago-gastric varices by surgical intervention, these procedures are hazardous and carry high operative mortality and morbidity. It is therefore justifiable to use a simpler and safer technique of oesophago-gastric tamponade before surgery is contemplated. The Sengstaken tri-lumen oesophageal tube has been in use for this purpose for many years but has recently been replaced by the Minnesota four-lumen tube. The latter is a complex tube which reaches into the stomach, where it is retained by a large balloon. This balloon is pulled up against the fundus of the stomach at the gastro-oesophageal junction. Just above the gastric balloon is a cylindrical balloon which compresses the lower one-third of the oesophagus. Two aspiration channels serve to decompress the stomach and oesophageal lumen above the oesophageal balloon. The latter channel is the most important modification of the Sengstaken tube, as it prevents accumulation of saliva above the oesophageal balloon, thus reducing the risk of pulmonary

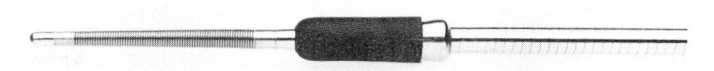

Fig.64 Photograph showing gripping element of Nottingham introducer in non-expanded positon (Key Med)

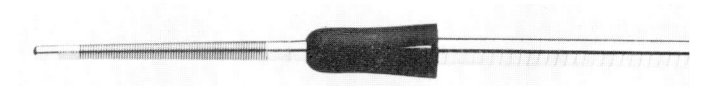

Fig.66 Key Med Nottingham oesophageal tube introducer set.

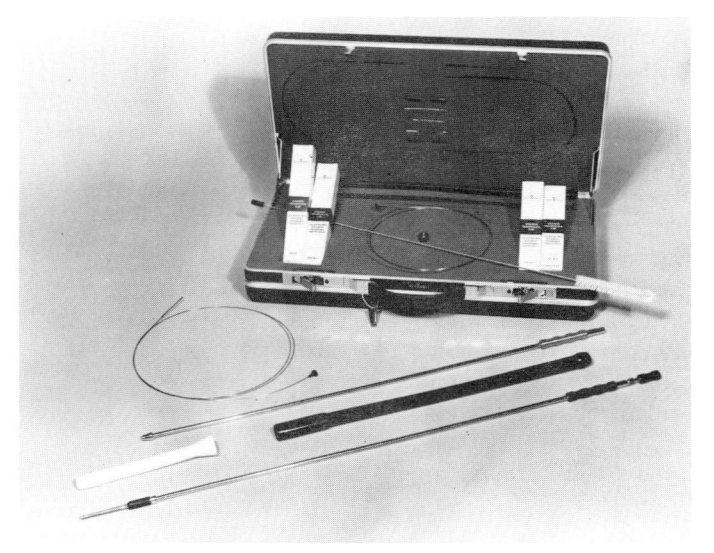

Fig.65 Photograph showing gripping element of Nottingham introducer in expanded position (Key Med)

aspiration. Before passing the tube, both balloons are inflated, using a mercury manometer to determine the pressure/volume relationship of each balloon. A nasogastric tube is passed into the stomach, and blood and clot lavaged. The tube is removed and the patient is positioned on a table with the head elevated at 45°. After removing all air from the balloons the tube is introduced pernasally into the posterior pharynx and, with the patient swallowing, passed to the 50 cm mark indicating that the distal end is in the stomach. Both the gastric and oesophageal lumen are aspirated. The gastric balloon is then inflated up to the volume of 400–500 ml. The tube is pulled back until resistance of the diaphragm is felt and it is then secured to the nose. The oesophageal balloon is inflated to a pressure of 35–45 mmHg. The oesophageal lumen is continuously aspirated using a low-suction pump and the gastric lumen is aspirated intermittently. After bleeding has stopped, the pressure of the oesophageal balloon should be reduced by 50 mmHg every three hours. Prolonged inflation of the balloon can produce pressure necrosis of the oesophageal wall and it should therefore be deflated after 24 hours of continuous compression for at least five minutes at regular intervals.

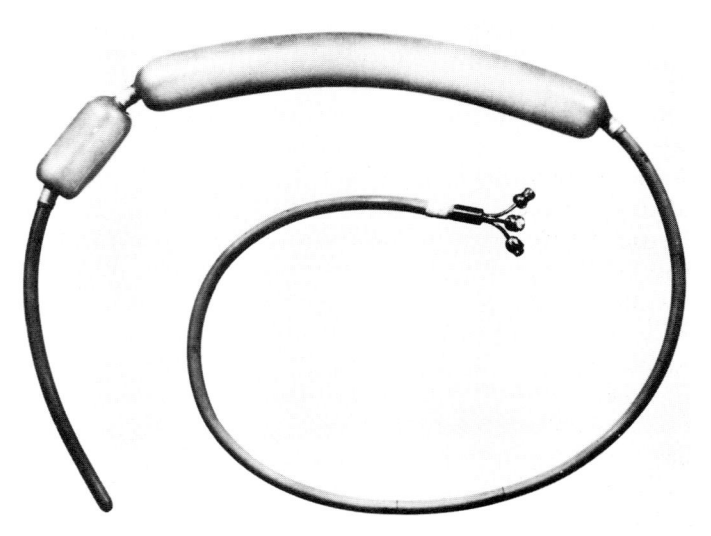

Fig.67 Sengstaken oesophageal tube

Symonds, C.J. (1855) A case of malignant stricture of the oesophagus illustrating the use of a new form of oesophageal catheter. *Transactions of the Clinical Society of London*, **28**, 155-158

Souttar, H.S. (1927) Treatment of carcinoma of the oesophagus based on 100 personal cases and 18 post-mortem reports. *British Journal of Surgery*, **15**, 76-91

Mousseau, M. *et al.* (1956) Place de l'intubation a demeure dans le traitement palliatif du coueur de l'oesophage. *Archives des Maladies de l'Appareil Digestif et de la Nutrition*, **45**, 208-214

Atkinson, M., Fergusson, R. and Parker, G.C. (1978) Tube introducer and modified Celestin tube for use in palliative intubation of oesophago-gastric neoplasms at fibreoptic endoscopy. *Gut*, **19**, 669-671

Atkinson, M. (1981) Intubation of oesophagogastric neoplasms. In: *Therapeutic Endoscopy* (ed. Bennett, J.R.), pp. 27-46. Chapman and Hall, London.

Edlich, R.F., Lande, A.J., Goodale, R.L. and Wangensteen, O.H. (1968) Prevention of aspiration pneumonia by continuous oesophageal aspiration during oesophagogastric tamponade and gastric cooling. *Surgery*, **64**, 405

5.3 Abdominal drains

Drains in abdominal surgery have been and remain a controversial subject. The question 'to drain or not to drain?' is being asked repeatedly. Although the use of drains for ascites was described by Celsus it was with the introduction of transperitoneal operations that drains became firmly established.

In the early stages drains were made of rubber wicks, gauze, or glass or silver tubes. In 1859 Chassaignac introduced a soft rubber tube drain and in 1882 Kehrer described a cigarette drain (gauze within a rubber sheath). In 1898 Keaton described the first suction drain.

The aim of the use of drains is the prevention of fluid collection within the abdominal cavity. Although their use is controversial, it can be said that drains should be used for the prevention of collection of fluid, prevention of generalised peritonitis, and obliteration of cavities. That every conceivable material has been used for their manufacture bears witness to the fact that there is no ideal abdominal drain. However, there is no doubt that most drains should be made of soft and non-irritant material, to minimise damage to intra-abdominal organs and to reduce inflammatory reaction to a minimum. In some cases a drain made of irritant material, such as rubber, is used deliberately to create a fibrous track. This applies to the drainage of chronic abscesses and bile ducts.

Drains are generally divided into non-suction and suction types. Non-suction drains provide an artificial track between the peritoneal cavity and the skin. Fluid drains either through the drain lumen (tube drain) or along its surface (corrugated drain) due to gravity and to the pressure differential between the inside and outside. The introduction of gauze into a tube drain introduces a capillary drainage effect. The Penrose drain, a tube drain made of latex rubber, is popular because it is soft, available in several sizes, and readily sterilised. Other tube drains are relatively rigid, ensuring that the lumen remains patent throughout their use. It is a common practice to cut out holes in the intra-abdominal portion of the tube drain in an attempt to increase the area of effective drainage. There is some evidence, however, that these holes soon become blocked by clot, fibrin and omentum. Corrugated drains allow drainage along the surface. They are effective but less manageable as the drainage fluid escapes on to the skin surface. The use of suction drains is controversial. They are tube drains to which suction is applied. The suction pressure can be considerable, as in the case of Red-i-vac drains, or small when suction pumps are used. High suction pressure undoubtedly leads to early obstruction of drain inlet holes, and consequently to ineffective or no drainage. Surrounding organs may also be easily damaged by the effect of suction. Their advantage is that they are closed drains and retrograde infection is less likely.

The disadvantages of continuous suction are avoided by the use of sump drains. These are hollow, rigid tubes under continuous suction with a separate air inlet, which allows the pressure to equalise within the suction lumen. These drains are particularly suitable for prolonged drainage of relatively large volumes of fluid, as in intestinal fistulas. The system remains a closed one with the addition of an air filter at the air inlet. The Shirley drain is probably the most versatile type of sump drain currently available. Quite apart from the fact that they may not always be effective, the use of drains is not without complications. Haemorrhage can occur from the drain wound and infection can be introduced by retrograde migration of bacteria. Incisional hernia can arise, especially if the stab wound is very large. One of the most serious complications is fistula formation due to pressure necrosis of the viscus. There is some evidence that the use of drains is associated with an increased incidence of anastomotic leakage after bowel anastomosis. This is probably due to the drain interposition between the anastomosis and omentum and intense inflammatory reaction at the anastomotic site. Drains are sometimes retained within the abdomen, mainly because of failure to secure them adequately. The last, but not the least, problem is the false sense of security when drains are used following surgery with inadequate haemostasis or unsatisfactory anastomosis.

Cerise, E.J. (1978) Drains in abdominal surgery: their use and abuse. In: *Practice of Surgery — Current Review* (ed. Ballinger, W.F.). Mosby, St. Louis.

Gunn, A.A. (1969) Abdominal drainage. *British Journal of Surgery*, 56, 274.

Duthie, H.L. (1972) Drainage of the abdomen. *New England Journal of Medicine*, 287, 1081.

Yates, J.L. (1905) An experimental study on the local effects of peritoneal drainage. *Surgery, Gynecology & Obstetrics*, 1, 473.

5.4 Chest drains

The purpose of a chest drain is to allow drainage of fluid from the pleural cavity as well as re-expansion of the lungs. Drains used following thoracic surgery are simply plastic or rubber tubes, with or without side holes in the intrapleural portion of the drain. They are all connected to a closed sterile system which allows fluid and air to drain in one direction only. In an emergency, the pneumothorax or haemothorax may have to be drained quickly, and drains are inserted percutaneously for this purpose. Prior to the introduction of disposable drains this was achieved with the aid of a trochar and cannula through which a piece of tubing was placed within the pleural cavity. The introduction of the Argyle pattern chest drain has simplified this procedure. The cannula is a transparent plastic tube with bevelled edges at the tip and 5 cm calibrations to determine the depth of insertion. Some tubes also have radio-opaque markers to make the drain radiologically visible. The sizes range from 10 to 32 FG. PVC material is less irritant to pleura than rubber and this is of advantage in the majority of cases. Within the cannula is a trochar metal needle which stiffens it and provides a sharp point, facilitating insertion through the chest wall. The trochar has a groove along its whole length to allow drainage of fluid and air prior to its removal from the cannula. On the proximal end of the trochar is a plastic ball handle to prevent injury to the operator's hand.

A convenient site must be selected prior to the drain insertion and this is chosen on radiological, clinical and anatomical grounds. In most cases the drain is inserted through the fourth interspace in the mid-axillary line. The procedure is carried out under local anaesthesia. After skin preparation and local anaesthetic infiltration the skin and tissues in the intercostal space are incised and a purse string suture is placed around the incision. The trochar and cannula are placed in the incision in contact with the upper border of the rib and directed towards the apex or base of the pleural cavity, as the case may be. Considerable pressure is required to penetrate the thoracic wall and sudden 'give' will indicate that the pleural cavity has been entered. The trochar is withdrawn, and the cannula temporarily clamped (except in tension pneumothorax) and secured to the skin. A connection is made with an underwater-seal bottle. The presence of bubbling air in the bottle on coughing and swinging water level indicate that the drain is within the pleural cavity. A chest X-ray is required to check the position of the drain.

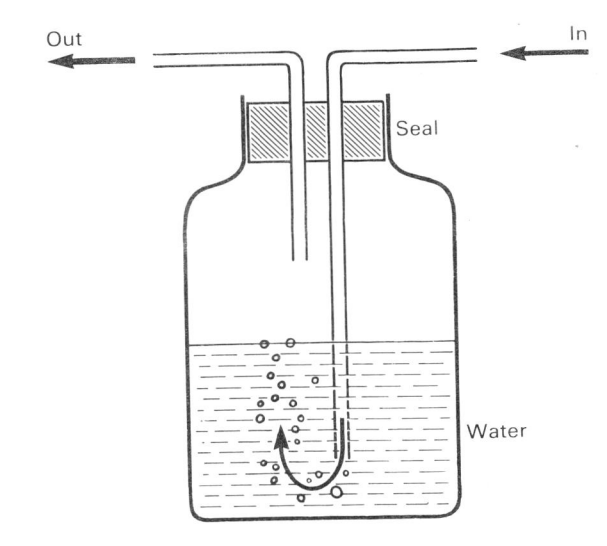

Fig.68 Underwater-seal bottle

Firman, R.K. and Welch, J.D. (1980) Insertion of a chest drain. *Update*, 1980, 481-486.

5.5 Urological catheters

Urological catheters are being increasingly used to decompress or splint any part of the urinary system. The Romans are known to have used urethral catheters with a plug of wool at the end which was pulled out with a thread after catheter insertion. The catheters were rigid and made of metal or horn and lubricated with an astringent. Fabricius described a catheter made of cloth mounted on a silver wire and impregnated with wax.

56 THERAPEUTIC INSTRUMENTS

Flexible catheters were first described at the end of the seventeenth century and the first rubber-covered catheter was introduced by Bernard in 1735. However, these catheters were unsuitable for prolonged usage, due to lack of elasticity in the cold and stickiness in hot weather. From the mid nineteenth century catheters were made of silver or steel. During this time it also became apparent that the male urethra was not right-angled and catheters were produced with less acute curves. It was not until recently that urethral catheters have been revolutionised by the introduction of modern materials and technology, making them less traumatic and safer. The self-retaining balloon catheter, designed by Foley, was originally designed to control haemorrhage after prostatectomy. It was first demonstrated by Foley in 1935. However, the design was first patented by P.A. Raiche of the Davol Rubber Company and Foley lost the subsequent law suit. The Foley catheter is a plastic two-lumen tube with an integral inflatable balloon. The balloon is inflated via a small valved channel. Modern urethral catheters, self-retaining or non-retaining, are made of materials which are the least irritant to the urethra. Silastic is the least irritant but it is soft and expensive. This material is particularly suitable for long-term catheterisation. Latex coated with polysiloxane elastomer is superior to latex alone but these catheters are thicker with a consequently smaller lumen.

Moreover, they are collapsible under suction and therefore less suitable where bladder washout is required. This problem can be avoided by using PVC catheters with a latex balloon (Simplastic), designed by J.G. Franklin in 1974. The advantage of PVC lies in its firmness, which avoids the need for

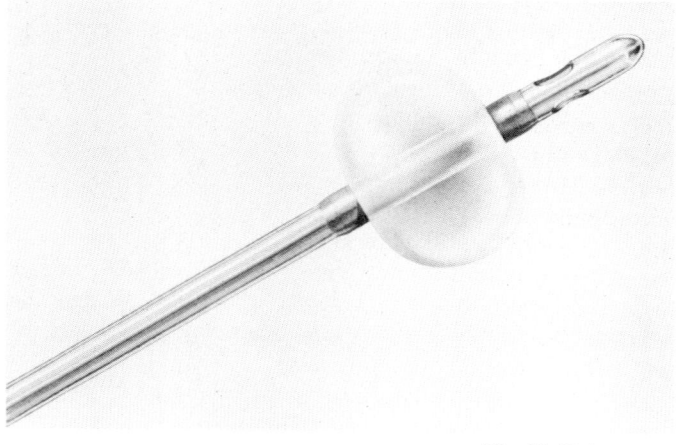

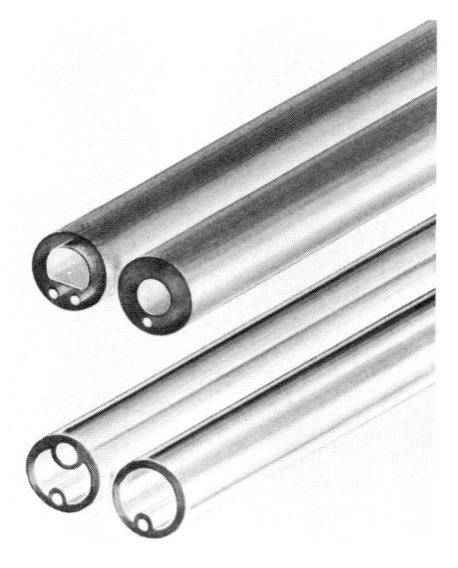

Fig.69 Foley balloon catheter (Franklin Medical)

Fig.70 Cross-section of urethral catheters (Franklin Medical)

catheter introducers, and yet, because of its thermoplasticity, the catheter softens at body temperature. Aspiration does not result in luminal collapse.

The choice of catheter tips is important. These can be straight or curved. Curved catheters are called coude and are specifically designed to pass the prostatic urethra distorted by prostatic enlargement. The Tiemann catheter has a stiff, pointed coude tip which is particularly suitable for the difficult prostatic urethra. Whistle-tipped catheters have a bevelled end which communicates with the main catheter lumen. They are suitable where clot retention is anticipated. Three-way catheters are designed for continuous irrigation. The additional small channel provides an inlet for irrigating fluid. The disadvantage of these catheters is that the addition of a third channel reduces the size of the main outflow lumen and consequently only large catheters provide satisfactory drainage. Urethral catheters are available in sizes 8–26 FG.

Suprapubic cystostomy is an alternative way of draining the urinary bladder. This can be carried out through a formal bladder exposure and any form of tube drain is satisfactory. The Malecot catheter is well suited for this purpose. It is a rubber or latex tube with two wings at the tip. These can be straightened over a wire introducer and are self-retaining. The de Pezzer catheter is based on a similar principle except that instead of wings it has a bulbous end which

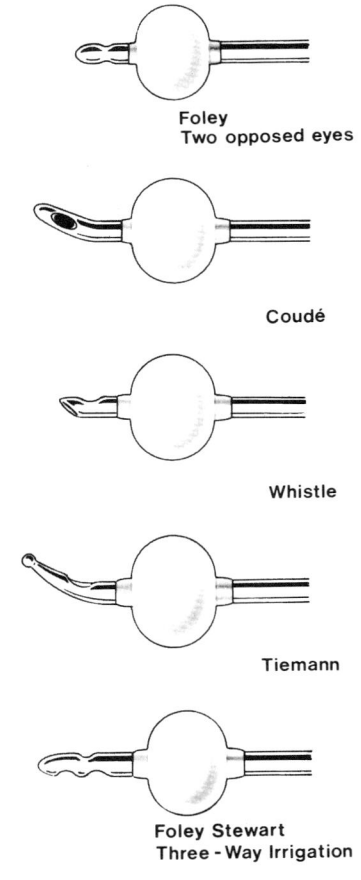

Fig.71 Urethral catheter tips (Franklin Medical)

Foley
Two opposed eyes

Coudé

Whistle

Tiemann

Foley Stewart
Three - Way Irrigation

can be straightened and recoils back when the wire introducer is removed. Percutaneous suprapubic cystostomy does not require a formal exposure of the bladder and is therefore indicated where cystostomy is a primary procedure. It can be safely carried out under local anaesthesia. The lower abdomen is shaved and suitably prepared. The position of the bladder is ascertained by percussion. Skin and subcutaneous tissues, including the bladder wall, are infiltrated in the midline and a small incision is made in the skin. The suprapubic trochar and cannula are pushed firmly into the wound and downward until the bladder is entered. The trochar is then removed, and the cannula secured to the skin and connected to a closed drainage system. Some percutaneous suprapubic catheters have inflatable balloons as an alternative to skin fixation. However, these catheters are stiff and large, making them uncomfortable for the patient.

Kidneys and ureters can now be drained percutaneously or endoscopically. Percutaneous drainage is based on the introduction of a flexible guide wire over which a suitable soft catheter is inserted. Ureters can be drained with fine self-retaining ureteric catheters. They can be inserted either percutaneously through the renal pelvis, peroperatively or endoscopically via the bladder. They are self-retaining by virtue of their curved ends, either J (Surgitek Double J) or pigtail shaped (Vance Products Inc.). Multiple drainage holes along the whole length of the catheter ensure satisfactory drainage. They are made of silicone or polyethylene. Endoscopically the ureteric orifice is identified and a taper-tip catheter passed into the renal pelvis under fluoroscopic control. The guide wire is introduced through the catheter and this is withdrawn. An appropriately sized double-ended pigtail catheter is passed over the guide wire, thus straightening both pigtail ends, and is advanced into the renal pelvis with the stent-pushing catheter. The guide wire is withdrawn and the coils form spontaneously in the renal pelvis and bladder. The catheter can be removed endoscopically using bladder biopsy forceps.

Zorgniotti, A.W. (1973) Frederick E.B. Foley: Early development of balloon catheter. *Urology*, **1**, 75-80.

Griffiths, D.A. and Shorey, B.A. (1976) Suprapubic cystostomy. *Hospital Update*, 1976, 537

Jones, P.A., Moxon, R.A., Pittam, M.R. and Edwards, L. (1983) Double-ended pigtail polyethylene stents in management of benign and malignant ureteric obstruction. *Journal of the Royal Society of Medicine*, **76**, 458.

5.6 Peritoneal dialysis catheters

Peritoneal dialysis is a well established procedure in acute renal failure. Patients with suspected intra-abdominal injury may benefit from diagnostic peritoneal lavage to avoid unnecessary laparotomy, especially if other injuries are present. Both procedures can be achieved by placing a catheter into the peritoneal cavity, allowing infusion and drainage of fluid.

The catheter consists of a cannula and trochar and connecting tubing with a shut-off mechanism and provision for injection of drugs. In contradistinction to most abdominal drains the cannula is semi-rigid, and is approximately 4 mm in diameter with a curved end. It has a large number of drainage holes along 10 cm of its distal end to facilitate drainage. The trochar is metal and pointed at one end with a plastic handle at the other. The connection tubing fits on to the cannula. The catheter can be inserted under local anaesthesia, usually in the midline below the umbilicus.

Prior to its insertion the bladder should be emptied of urine to avoid its accidental damage. The skin is incised down to and including the linea alba and the trochar with cannula is inserted into the incision. The tip of the catheter should be aimed towards the left or right pelvic gutter. There is a slight 'give' when the cannula punctures the peritoneum, at which stage the trochar should be partially withdrawn to prevent damage to the bowel. The cannula is then advanced into the peritoneal cavity, the trochar removed and the connection tubing attached.

The main hazard of this procedure is a penetrating injury to viscus and major pelvic blood vessels. However, these complications are surprisingly rare.

Bailey, M.J. (1978) Peritoneal lavage in blunt abdominal trauma. *Update*, November 1978, 749-755.

5.7 Peritoneo-venous shunt

Until recently the only effective treatment for intractable ascites in portal hypertension was some form of portacaval shunt. This operation has a high operative mortality and the surviving patient runs the risk of encephalopathy and hepatic failure. Continuous or intermittent external drainage of ascites is also unsatisfactory.

In 1974 Le Veen introduced a new technique of slow peritoneo-venous drainage known as Le Veen shunt. This consists of a proximal peritoneal tube, a shunt valve and a distal venous tube. The shunt valve is a one-way diaphragm valve which opens when the intraperitoneal pressure is 3 cm of water higher than the central and intra-thoracic pressures. This occurs mainly during inspiration when central venous pressure falls and intra-abdominal pressure increases.

The valve is placed between the peritoneum and abdominal muscles in the right hypochondrium. The peritoneal tube is inserted intra-abdominally and tied with a purse-string in the peritoneum. The venous tube is pulled through a stab wound in the abdominal muscles. The muscles are tightly closed over the valve to prevent leakage of ascites. The ipsilateral internal jugular vein is exposed in the neck and the venous tube is pulled into the wound subcutaneously. The tube is then passed into the jugular vein through a venotomy and secured, the proximal end of the vein having previously been tied. The tube end should lie in the superior vena cava.

Post-operatively it is necessary to produce maximum diuresis and the extent of haemodilution must be monitored with frequent haematocrit and serum potassium measurement. The shunt is contraindicated in patients with liver failure, peritonitis and recent gastrointestinal bleeding. The complications include infection, subcutaneous bleeding, leakage of ascitic fluid and shunt failure.

Le Veen, H.H., Christoudias, G., Ip, M., Luft, R., Falk, G. and Grosberg, S. (1974) Peritoneo-venous shunting for ascites. *Annals of Surgery*, **180**, 580-591.

Le Veen, H.H. and Wapnick, S. (1975) Operative details of continuous peritoneo-venous shunt for ascites. *Bulletin de la Sôcieté Internationale de Chirurgie*, **6**, 579-582.

5.8 Biliary drains

The most well known biliary drain is the T-tube for decompression of the common bile duct after surgical exploration. The Kerr pattern tube is a T-shaped tubular drain in various sizes. The cross-bar is placed into the common bile duct and bile is allowed to drain out through the long segment brought out through the abdominal wall. Some T-tubes, such as the Maingot, have part of the circumference of the cross-bar removed to reduce obstruction to bile duct flow and also to facilitate its removal.

T-tubes are traditionally made out of latex to stimulate peritoneal reaction with formation of a fibrous track. Silicone T-tubes have been introduced but these are unpopular because of reports of biliary peritonitis following their removal.

Percutaneous transhepatic cholangiography for obstructive jaundice has been in use for more than 20 years. A sheathed needle was used for this purpose and this procedure was not uncommonly accompanied by biliary peritonitis requiring urgent surgical intervention.

In 1974 Okuda described a fine needle technique (Chiba) which proved to be safer. Therapeutic percutaneous drainage of obstructed biliary tract was first described in 1952 by Carter and Saypole. Since then it has become possible not only to place catheters within the biliary tree to allow decompression but also, via the same route, to dilate strictures and insert endoprosthesis and allow biopsy.

The fine needle is introduced through lateral approach and dye is injected until the large right hepatic duct is entered. A sheathed needle is then introduced into the large duct, as outlined by contrast medium, and as soon as bile flows freely a guide wire with a J tip is passed into the duct. A catheter then may be advanced over the guide wire. The wire may be passed through a stricture and a ring catheter, very much like urinary pigtail catheters, or an endoprosthesis can be inserted over the wire for internal splinting. Endoprostheses are fairly large and stiff and strictures may have to be dilated prior to their insertion.

The complications associated with this technique are mostly due to bile leakage, cholangitis with septicaemia, haemobilia and puncture of adjacent organs.

Carter, R.F. and Saypole, G.M. (1952) Transabdominal cholangiography. *Journal of the American Medical Association*, **148**, 253.

Irving, J.D. (1981) Relief of biliary obstruction. *British Journal of Hospital Medicine*, 1981, 329-338.

Okuda, R. *et al.* (1974) Non-surgical percutaneous transhepatic cholangiography. *American Journal of Digestive Disease*, **19**, 21-36.

5.9 Tracheostomy and endotracheal tubes

Tracheostomy has been practised for hundreds of years for the relief of upper respiratory obstruction. Before the introduction of proper surgical technique and tracheostomy tubes, it carried a very high mortality. Since the advent of modern endotracheal tubes and ventilation its use has been limited to cases requiring prolonged ventilation: in major head and neck surgery, in patients with deficient swallowing reflex and in some cases of laryngitis and epiglottitis. There is virtually no place for 'emergency' tracheostomy in hospital practice.

The most well known tracheostomy tube is the Negus silver (KCH pattern) type. The tube set consists of the curved tube with a recessed valved inner tube and a plain inner tube with a pilot. The pilot, or obturator, is used during the tube insertion. It is removed after secure placement of the tube into the trachea. The inner tube is removed for cleaning, avoiding the need for the removal of the tracheostomy tube from the trachea. It is longer than the outer

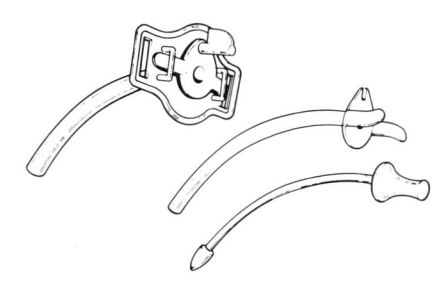

Fig.72 Chevalier–Jackson tracheostomy tube (Downs)

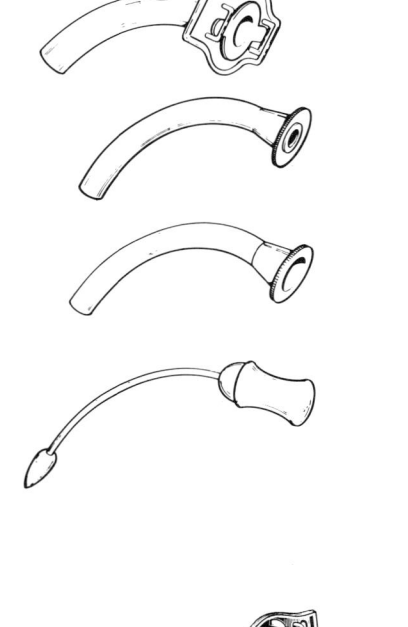

Fig.73 Negus tracheostomy tube (Downs)

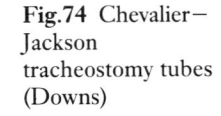

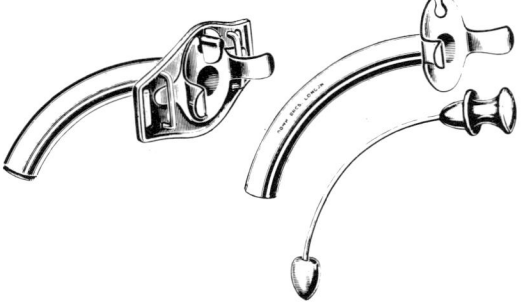

Fig.74 Chevalier–Jackson tracheostomy tubes (Downs)

tube so that the latter cannot remain obstructed when the inner tube is removed for cleaning. The valved inner tube is used in patients with permanent tracheostomy to prevent emission of mucus during coughing and to improve their speech.

The flange on the end is used for securing the tube. Modern tracheostomy tubes are made of plastic material and are manufactured with or without an inflatable cuff. The cuff is used in patients on respirators and needs to be inflated and deflated at regular intervals to prevent pressure necrosis to the trachea. Plastic tubes are softer, less irritant, sterile and disposable.

Without endotracheal tubes modern anaesthesia would be unthinkable. The first endotracheal tube for ventilation of lungs was described by Alexander Monroe in 1774. Its use has been firmly established for the last sixty years. The traditional tubes of the Magill pattern are made of red mineralized rubber. Modern tubes are made of plastic and are disposable.

Except for the smallest they all have an inflatable cuff near the distal tip to protect the lower respiratory tract from soiling as well as providing an air-tight seal for assisted ventilation. In order to provide some indication of the degree of cuff inflation, the cuff tube is provided with a pilot cuff just distal to its syringe connection.

The tubes are made in various sizes, indicated by numbers. Each number refers to the internal diameter of the tube in millimetres. The size of the tube used depends on the patient's sex and age. In children the following formula is used: age (years) + 4.5 = internal diameter in millimetres. In adults the average size is 8.5 for females and 9.5 for males.

Dunkin, L.J. (1980) How to intubate. *British Journal of Hospital Medicine*, January 1980, 77-80.
Jones, D.F. (1979) Endotracheal intubations. *Hospital Update*, December 1979, 1107-1117.
Griffith, D.A. and Shorley, B.A. (1976) Emergency tracheostomy. *Hospital Update*, 1976, 311-315.
Griffith, I.P. (1976) Tracheostomy. *British Journal of Hospital Medicine*, 1976, 76-86.
Feldman, S.A. and Crawley, B.E. (eds) *Tracheostomy and Assisted Ventilation*, 2nd edn. Edward Arnold, London.

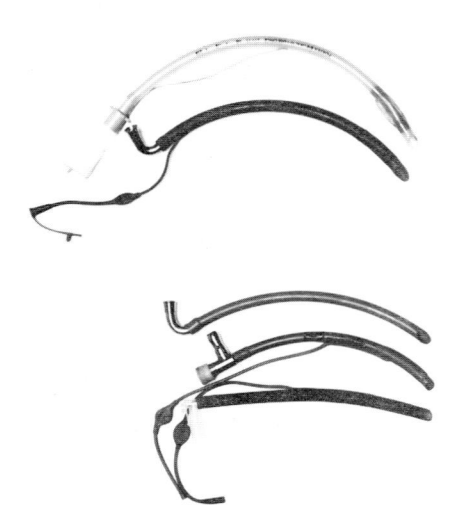

Fig.75 Endotracheal tubes

Chapter 6

Diathermy, Cryosurgery, Ultrasound, Dornier Lithotripter

6.1 Diathermy
6.2 Cryosurgery
6.3 Laser
6.4 Dornier extracorporeal shock wave lithotripsy

6.1 Diathermy

Undoubtedly diathermy is one of the most important technical innovations of modern surgery. The term diathermy was coined by Nagelschmidt in 1909. It is a technique of coagulating or cutting tissues by means of an electric current, which, if allowed to flow between two points in the body tissues, results in a temperature increase at the point of contact.

Electrocautery, on the other hand, produces heat to coagulate or fulgurate by means of a current flowing through a resistor. It utilizes small voltage and high current.

In diathermy the rise in temperature depends on the electrical resistance of tissues and the strength of the current. If a continuous current is used a muscle twitch is produced, and sufficiently rapid switching on and off produces tetany, that is, a progressive muscle contraction. Tetany is abolished by a sufficiently high-frequency current, which blocks conduction through nerves. Modern diathermy machines utilise frequencies between 300 kHz and 5 MHz.

If one point of contact is large, the heat is dissipated over this large area and the rise in temperature is insignificant. A small point of contact on the other hand will produce a very large temperature rise, resulting in coagulation or cutting.

With increasing current the temperature increases until an arc is struck, resulting in cutting with little heating of surrounding tissues. A lower current produces coagulation.

Diathermy generators produce currents at frequencies between 300 kHz and 5 MHz. There are two types of diathermy current generators.

The spark-gap generator is said to produce the best coagulation and consists of a capacitor which

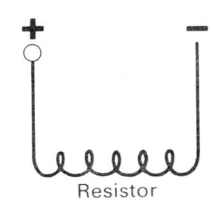

Fig.76 Electrocautery circuit

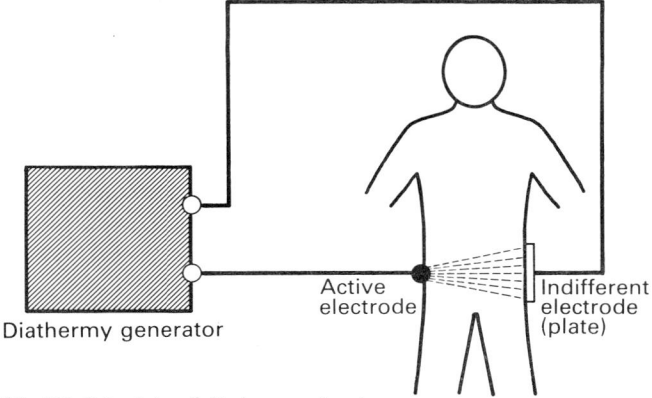

Fig.77 Principle of diathermy circuit

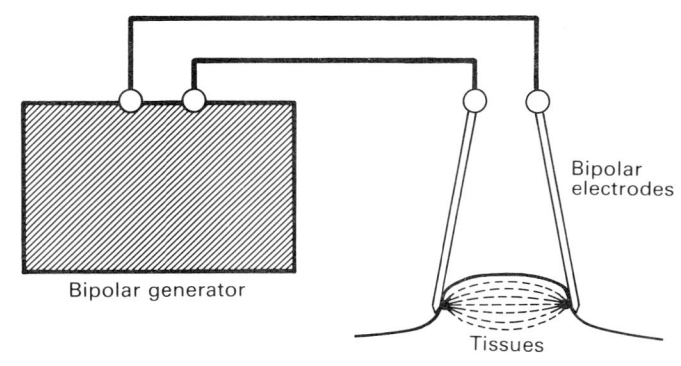

Fig.78 Principle of bipolar diathermy

discharges through a coil and spark gap. This circuit produces a series of high-frequency damped oscillations.

The valve circuit generator produces a current suitable for cutting. A high-voltage current at 50 Hz frequency is passed through an anode valve, producing an oscillating current at 2–5 MHz frequency while the anode is positive. During the negative phase no discharge takes place. Thus high-frequency waves are produces 50 times per second.

A combination of these currents results in a 'blended current'; this both coagulates and cuts. Newer generators utilise transistorised circuits which are capable of producing a wide range of high-frequency wave forms. They are small and portable.

The effectiveness of diathermy also depends on the conductivity of tissues. Fat, for example, is a poor conductor. The size of the electrode has an effect of the amount of heat produced; the smaller the electrode, the higher is the temperature at the point of contact.

The use of diathermy carries the risk of accidental burns to the patient and the surgeon.

If the current is allowed to return to earth through a small contact, rather than through the large indifferent electrode, the tissues in contact are heated to the same extent as the active electrode. If the large indifferent electrode is properly attached such accidental burning cannot occur.

When the plate wire is broken, or not plugged into the machine, the current tries to find its way to earth and any contact of the patient's body with metal parts of the table will complete the circuit. ECG electrodes are another source of potential earthing contact and there should therefore be sufficient resistance between the electrodes and the body to prevent a leak of high-frequency current.

Modern diathermy machines have safety devices which give warning when the current is poor or incomplete. Others incorporate a small capacitor between the plate and the patient; the current flows directly to earth and a diathermy current is not established.

Patients with pacemakers are at special risk when exposed to diathermy. Demand pacemakers can be inappropriately stimulated by the diathermy current and the pacemaker circuiting can be damaged, resulting in cardiac dysrhythmia.

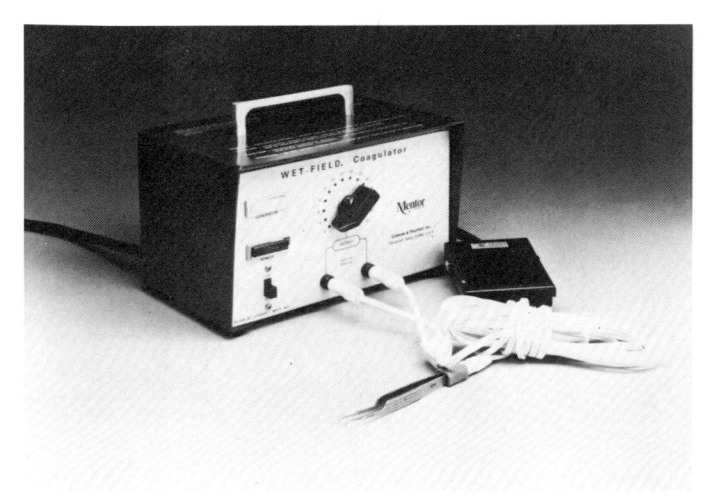

Fig.79 Wet-field bipolar generator (Codman)

Blandy, J.P. (1978) *Transurethral Resection*, 2nd edn. Pitman Medical, London.

Mitchell, J.P. and Lumb, G.N. (1966) *A Handbook of Surgical Diathermy*. John Wright, Bristol

Dobbie, A.K. (1969) The electrical aspects of surgical diathermy. *Biomedical Engineering*, 4, 206.

Mitchell, J.P. and Dobbie, A.K. (1976) Surgical diathermy in urological practice. In: *Scientific Foundations of Urology* (ed. Williams, D.I. and Chisholm, G.D.) Heinemann, London.

6.2 Cryosurgery

Cryosurgery is the technique of destruction of living tissues by controlled cooling.

Although water and ice have been known to relieve pain for many centuries it was not until 1851 that James Arnot of the Middlesex Hospital in London described the therapeutic use of freezing mixture ($-20°C$) of salt and ice. He applied this mixture for various ailments including breast carcinoma and carcinoma of the cervix. He noted that the freezing effect of this mixture had an anaesthetic as well as a haemostatic effect.

During the early part of the twentieth century, liquid air and CO_2 snow were used therapeutically for superficial skin lesions, mainly in dermatology. Liquid nitrogen replaced CO_2 snow but its application was still unsatisfactory, mainly because of its uncontrollable effect.

In 1962 Irvine Cooper of New York described a probe which was cooled by circulating liquid nitrogen to $-196°C$. It was vacuum insulated, except for the tip. He used it in neurosurgery for Parkinson's disease, as well as for the treatment of a variety of malignant tumours. Since then technical innovation has provided us with simpler and much more flexible probes, allowing a greater degree of controlled tissue destruction.

The effect of cryosurgery is a uniform injury to living cells, which eventually die from the effects of freezing. It is not known precisely why this uniform death should occur, since tissue cultures may survive cooling to very low temperatures.

It has been suggested that cell death is caused by the formation of intracellular ice crystals with resulting cell dehydration and denaturation of cell proteins. The second phase of cellular destruction is due to the obliteration of microcirculation within the frozen tissue. No cells can survive ischaemic infarction, regardless of whether they are resistant to cold. This would explain why cells taken from frozen tissue after thawing survive, whereas those taken from the same tissue after 24 hours are dead. The theory that ischaemia is the final cause of cell death is also supported by the observation that cell death is uniform throughout the cryolesion, despite a gradient of decreasing temperature from the centre of the lesion.

The size of the cryolesion and its growth are related to factors such as the probe size, its temperature and the duration of freezing.

The growth of the cryolesion from the central freezing point is directly related to the ice/water boundary. The lesion eventually assumes the shape of a sphere. The relationship between the size of the lesion and the size of the probe and its temperature is a direct one. However, the relationship between the size of the lesion and the duration of freezing is logarithmic. This only applies to one constant application. Several successive applications will increase the volume of frozen tissue so that the overall effect is greater than that of one continuous application of the same duration. It is thought that this is due to an increase in thermo-conductivity of tissues previously exposed to freezing.

For practical purposes, in surface cyrosurgery the extent of tissue destruction is related to the visible colour change of tissue. The simplest form of cryosurgery is a topical application of a cotton wool ball attached to a wooden stick, dipped in liquid nitrogen. Alternatively, a copper stick with an insulated handle may be used. This system is inefficient and requires a supply of liquid nitrogen, which readily evaporates. The temperature achieved is $-190°C$. This temperature cannot be used in body cavities. Surrounding tissues have to be protected from contact with the liquid.

Probes utilising liquid nitrogen ($-190°C$) or liquid nitrous oxide ($-90°C$) require vacuum insulation and are therefore expensive. The flow of liquid to the tip can be regulated, thus allowing for control of temperature. Thermocouples can indicate the tip temperature. Some probes have a heating coil built into the probe, which allows the tip to be rewarmed.

Gas probes are based on the Joul–Thompson effect of expanding gas taking up heat from its surroundings. Nitrous oxide is used most commonly, at a pressure of approximately 50 kg cm^{-2}, producing a tip temperature of $-75°C$.

These probes are not as powerful as those utilising liquid nitrogen and consequently are less haemostatic. They will stick to moist tissues when warm and this may facilitate removal of some lesions. This property depends on the size of ice crystals and appears to be temperature limited. No adhesion occurs beyond $-80°C$.

The tip has to be rewarmed to allow the probe to be removed and this is done either by an electric coil or by a large volume of warm gas passed down the probe. These probes are more portable and less expensive.

Cryosurgery is used in a variety of conditions. It can be used to advantage for biopsy, and the reader is referred to Chapter 3.

Cryosurgery is particularly suitable for the treatment of a variety of benign and malignant lesions. Some lesions such as polyps, verrucas, and squamous cell and basal cell carcinomas of the skin are particularly suitable. In some malignant tumours palliation by cryosurgery has obvious advantages over other conventional treatment, especially since no anaesthesia is required and haemostasis is excellent.

Cryosurgery is also gaining popularity in ENT surgery for tonsilectomy, nasal surgery and oral tumours.

Holder, H.B. (ed.) (1975) *Practical Cryosurgery*. Pitman Medical, Tunbridge Wells.
Lloyd-Williams, L. (1978) In: *Cryosurgery and Its Applications in Current Surgical Practice*, Vol 2. (ed. Hadfield, J. and Hobsley, M.). Edward Arnold, London.

6.3 Laser

Laser is an acronym for 'light amplification by stimulated emission of radiation'.

Its power is derived from a beam of light of uniform wavelength which, on contact with an absorptive surface, liberates heat. Tissues exposed to this light beam coagulate or are evaporated.

In 1917 Einstein published the concept of stimulated emission. It was not until 1958 that the principles of microwave amplification by stimulated emission of radiation (maser) were described.

The first laser was introduced in 1960 by Maiman, who was able to produce a visible stimulated emission by exciting a ruby rod with a flashing white light. The first gas laser using helium and neon was demonstrated in 1961 by Javan. Since then different media have been used, solid and gaseous, each with different wavelengths and different physical properties.

Laser wavelengths not only cover the visible portion of the electromagnetic spectrum but also infra-red and ultraviolet portions of the spectrum.

An atom in its resting, or ground, state is capable of becoming excited by absorption of energy, whether optical, electric or thermal. The atom will then return to its ground state and liberate the absorbed energy — spontaneous emission of radiation. When an excited atom returns to the ground state after interaction with radiation of a wavelength which corresponds to the absorption energy wavelenth, two waves of the same wavelength are produced, in phase with each other and travelling in the same direction — stimulated emission of radiation. To produce a lasting action, more atoms must be in an excited state than at the ground state.

The basic laser consists of a tube containing the active medium, for instance a gas, which can undergo stimulated emission. At each end of the tube are concave mirrors, one of which totally reflects the energy. The opposite mirror is only partially

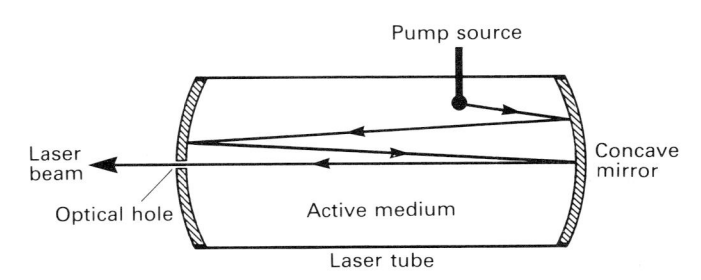

Fig.80 Principle of laser generation

reflective and thus is capable of transmitting part of the total energy. The initiating energy is imparted by the pump in the form of thermal, electric or light energy. The light created by spontaneous radiation will travel in all directions. Most of this radiation will be dissipated as heat. A small fraction of the radiation will travel along the laser tube. It is this radiation that will interact with excited atoms of the medium to produce stimulated emission of radiation. The energy thus produced is reflected by tube mirrors and amplified. Some of the energy escapes through the partially reflective mirror as a laser beam.

The light generated by laser can take the form of a continuous wave or multiple pulses. The pulsed laser beam has higher energy than continuous wave laser. If a fast shutter is interposed between the medium and the mirror, the energy builds up with the shutter closed and can be discharged by opening the shutter. This results in pulses of energy of short duration and high intensity — Q switching.

The effect of the laser beam on tissues depends on its spectrum, energy and tissue absorption. Currently there are three main types of laser used in surgery: CO_2, argon and Neodymium YAG.

CO_2 laser uses a mixture of CO_2 and nitrogen. The active medium is CO_2, and nitrogen acts to transfer energy from the pump to CO_2 molecules. The CO_2 molecule is brought down to the resting state by collision with helium atoms. Its emission is in the middle of the infrared spectrum (10.6 μm) and is well absorbed by water. The cells are vapourised and the latent heat transfers to adjacent cells. The adjacent area of damage is thus small, in spite of local rise of temperature to around 100°C. CO_2 laser is used for incisions or ablation of tissue by vapourisation. The laser beam can be delivered via an operating microscope or through a series of articulated mirrors.

Argon laser utilises argon gas as the active medium and an electric current as a pump. The light is in the visible green wavelength (0.5 μm) and is capable of producing relatively little energy. It is largely absorbed by haemoglobin and its main effect on tissues is coagulation. For this reason argon laser is used to seal blood vessels, haemangiomas and other skin lesions. Its main advantage is that it can be delivered via flexible fibre-optic rods and can thus be used in conjunction with flexible endoscopes.

Neodymium − yttrium − aluminium − garnet (YAG) laser is a solid state laser which utilises a krypton or xenon lamp as a pump. It produces an invisible beam of light (1.06 μm) and is capable of generating four times as much energy as argon laser. Although it is less strongly absorbed by haemoglobin than argon laser its main effect is coagulation. It too can be transmitted via flexible quartz fibres.

Laser has obvious advantages over diathermy, cryoprobe or even the scalpel. It is accurate, coagulates small vessels as it cuts, and is clean. It is, however, very expensive and clumsy. Currently it is used mainly for treatment of superficial skin lesions and in the gastrointestinal tract for bleeding and treatment of vascular lesions.

Because of its potential advantages laser will no doubt become a standard instrument for the surgeon of the future.

Maiman, T.H. (1980) Stimulated optical radiation in ruby. *Nature, London*, **187**, 493.
Cochrane, J.P.S. (1981) The use of lasers in general surgery. *Hospital Update*, February 1981, 91-99.
Vallon, A.G. (1982) Lasers and fibreoptic endoscopy. *British Journal of Hospital Medicine*, 1982, 175-179.
Dixon, J.A. (ed.) (1983) *Surgical Application of Lasers*. Year Book, Chicago.

6.4 Dornier extracorporeal shock wave lithotripsy

The recent introduction of Dornier kidney lithotripsy, percutaneous lithotripsy and rigid ureteroscopy means that open renal and ureteric surgery for stones may soon become a rarity.

The basic principle of shock-wave lithotripsy is the generation of shock waves which are precisely directed to the stone by means of two image-intensifier cameras. The shock waves are produced by an underwater spark discharge between two electrodes situated in an ellipsoidal reflector. They are generated in a medium which has similar acoustic properties to body tissues, namely water. The ellipsoidal reflector serves to reflect the waves in such a manner that they can be concentrated into a small area. The waves are then coupled to the medium and reflected to a focal point.

A portion of the shock wave entering a stone is absorbed because of a sudden change in acoustic resistance. Part of the shock wave is reflected by the stone. A portion of the penetrating

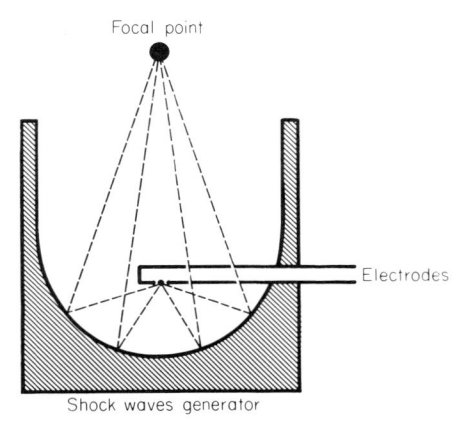

Fig.81 Shock wave generator

Fig.82 Effect of shock waves on stone

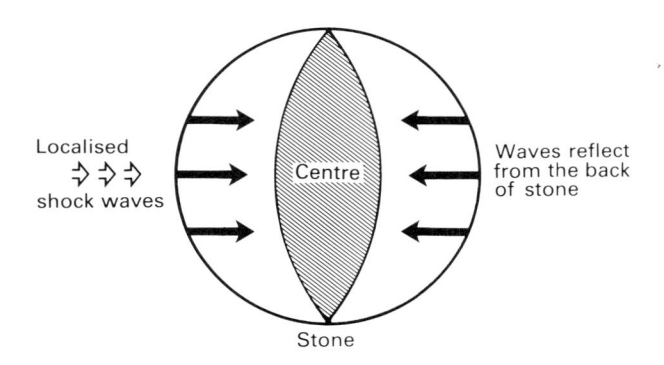

70 THERAPEUTIC INSTRUMENTS

wave is reflected from the opposite surface of the stone and this again leads to a build up of forces which shatter this segment of the stone, leaving the centre unaffected. A series of shock waves then eventually leads to complete disintergration.

The Dornier lithotripter is composed of a shock wave generator, coupling tub and frame, location system and patient-positioning system. The shock waves are produced in an ellipsoidal reflector between two electrodes immersed in water. The coupling medium is specially treated water, contained in a stainless steel tub.

The location system consists of two independent X-ray tubes which are aimed in such a way that their beams intersect in the second focus of the reflection. The X-ray cameras are placed exactly in the line of each X-ray beam and the picture is displayed on a monitor. The patient-positioning hydraulic system allows the adjustment of the kidney stone into the focal point of the shock wave reflection.

The results of this technique of kidney stone disintegration are encouraging, with better than 90% therapeutic success. There have been no reports of organ damage. A small percentage of patients experience a post-operative colic due to the passage of stone particles through the ureter.

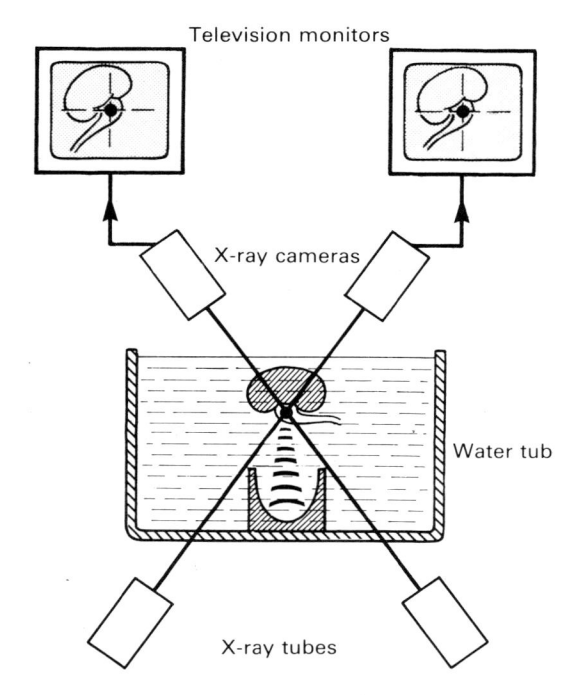

Fig.83 Dornier lithotripter

Chaussy, C.H., Brendel, W. and Schmiedt, E. (1980) Extracorporeally induced destruction of kidney stones by shock waves. *Lancet*, Dec 13, 1980, 1265-1268.

Chaussy, C.H., Schmiedt, E., Jocham, D., Brendel, W., Forssmann, B. and Walther, W. (1982) First clinical experience with extracorporeally induced destruction of kidney stones by shock waves. *Journal of Urology*, **127**, 417-420.

Chapter 7

Sterilisation, Sutures, Gloves, Implants

7.1 Sterilisation and disinfection
7.2 Surgical suture
7.3 Surgical gloves
7.4 Implants

7.1 Sterilisation and disinfection

There is no doubt that the introduction of general anaesthesia and antiseptics into surgery in the second part of the nineteenth century were the most important landmarks in the evolution of modern surgical practice.

Although the contributions of Semmelweiss and Holmes should not be forgotten, it was Lord Lister who developed the principles of antisepsis. He was the first to use carbolic acid spray during operations, resulting in a significant reduction of infection which, at that time, was the major cause of post-operative death.

Gradually, it was realised that in order to reduce post-operative infection it was necessary to use a sterile operating environment, as well as sterile instruments.

Sterilisation is a method of destroying all organisms, including spores. Disinfection, on the other hand, destroys only living organisms.

Asepsis is a technique of preventing access of organisms into the patient's uninfected tissues.

Heat is a physical form of disinfection. Hot air is inefficient, unless it reaches a temperature of 160°C and is circulated. Boiling, pasteurisation and tyndallisation provide moist heat, which is more useful because it is effective at lower temperatures and over a shorter period of time. Boiling for 10 minutes will not destroy spores but will destroy hepatitis virus.

Pasteurisation is achieved by heating at 63°C for 30 minutes or 72°C for 20 seconds. Again this process does not destroy spores or hepatitis virus but is suitable for some delicate instruments which cannot withstand boiling. Tyndallisation refers to steaming of a solution for 20 minutes every 24 hours for three consecutive days. This process will kill spores. The most important process of sterilisation in operating theatres is undoubtedly autoclaving. The principle of autoclaving is based on the fact that with increasing pressure the boiling point of water is raised. At a pressure of 15 psi the boiling point is raised to 121°C. Materials exposed to steam at this temperature for 15 minutes will be sterilised. At higher temperatures this process is more rapid.

Steam is preferable to dry heat because it acts by denaturing enzymes and proteins, penetrates better and as it condenses releases latent heat resulting in reduction in the volume of steam. This negative pressure effect draws in more steam. Steam has to be dry, free from air and close to the point of condensation. The autoclave is a steriliser with steam under pressure.

Modern autoclaves use a combination of a vacuum and high pressure. Prior to the introduction of steam the container is subjected to a vacuum and then steam is introduced at a pressure of 30 psi. At 134°C the process of autoclaving is over in three minutes.

The efficiency of autoclaving can be tested by a thermocouple, Browne's tubes or autoclave tape. Browne's tubes contain a chemical indicator which turns green at a specific temperature. Autoclave tapes are printed with heat-sensitive ink. Autoclaving is suitable for surgical instruments, dressings, drapes and gowns.

Gamma and beta ionising radiation is used commercially for sterilisation of disposable equipment which is unsuitable for autoclaving.

Clinical disinfectants are numerous and can be divided into inorganic and organic. They should be non-toxic, hypoallergic, non-irritating and effective against a wide range of organisms and spores. They should not be inactivated by tissues and organic materials.

Iodine and chlorine are representative of inorganic disinfectants. Tincture of iodine contains 25% iodine, potassium iodine and 90% ethanol. Although it is a good disinfectant it is irritating to exposed tissues, allergenic and stains badly. Povidone-iodine is a solution in a non-ionic detergent. Although not as effective as the tincture it is said to be less allergenic. Chlorine is supplied as hypochlorite or eusol (short for Edinburgh University Solution), which is a solution of chlorinated lime with boric acid.

Organic disinfectants are represented by alcohols, aldehydes, phenols and cationic surface-active agents. The most well known aldehyde is formalin, a solution of formaldehyde. It is slow in action, penetrates poorly, is sensitising and has an irritating odour. Dettol is the best known of phenols and is least irritant. It is, however, easily inactivated by organic matter. Chlorhexidine (Hibitane) is widely used for skin disinfection. It is active against most bacteria in solution in both water and alcohol. Hexacholorphane is insoluble in water or alcohol and is used in soap form. It is poorly active against Gram-negative bacteria, especially *Pseudomonas*. It is particularly good for eliminating staphylococci from the skin. Cetrimide is a cationic surface agent which acts by dissociating into large cations and small anions when in aqueous solution. It is only moderately bactericidal against Gram-positive organisms and ineffective against Gram-negative organisms. However, it is non-toxic and non-irritating.

Some gaseous compounds are suitable for sterilisation. Ethylene oxide boils at 12°C and is very effective against bacteria and spores, penetrates well and is odourless and non-toxic. However, it is inflammable and explosive, although less so if used with CO_2. This process of sterilisation takes 18 hours at 25°C and is therefore used for materials which cannot be autoclaved or where ionising radiation is not available.

Walter, J.B. and Israel, M.S. (1974) *The Principles of Disinfection in General Pathology*, 4th edn., pp. 637-643. Churchill Livingstone, Edinburgh.

7.2 Surgical suture

The first known documentation of sutures is found in the Egyptian medical writings of 4000 years ago. They describe linen threads and animal tendons for both ligating and suturing. In India, surgeons used animal tendons, leather strips and horse hair some 3000 years ago. Catgut was described in the first century AD. Silk has been in use for over 2000 years and is mentioned in the writings of Galen.

Over the last 20 years there has been a revolutionary change in the manufacture and sterilisation of sutures, and new synthetic materials have been introduced.

Suture materials are divided into absorbable and non-absorbable. Catgut is an absorbable material still widely used. It is made from submucosa of the proximal small intestine. It was Lister, who, while searching for a method of sterilising catgut, discovered that chromium sulphate hardened catgut to such an extent that the gut did not suffer from the softening action of carbolic acid solution. This was the beginning of chromicised catgut as we know it today.

Until recently catgut was placed in glass tubes and immersed for 24 hours in an antiseptic solution, such as formalin and alcohol, carbolic acid or 20% alcoholic iodine. In order to improve its handling characteristics catgut had to be kept in fluid prior to use. Boilable catgut was dehydrated and immersed in a solvent of high boiling point. The containers could therefore be heat sterilised. The disadvantage of treating catgut in such a way was that it became brittle and hard. To make catgut more flexible it had to be washed in alcohol and sterile water. This resulted in a material of varying strength and softness. Non-boilable catgut, on the other hand, was immersed in an alcoholic solution and was not suitable for heat sterilisation.

Currently catgut is produced from strips of sheep gut submucosa, which is subjected to mechanical cleaning so that the final product consists of pure collagen. The ribbons are then twisted together and chromed, if desired, dried under tension and polished. Sterilisation is achieved by ethylene oxide or gamma radiation and the product is packed in fluid for pliability. Tensile strength of plain catgut is lost within eight days; chromic catgut lasts about twice as long. Catgut also has poor knot-holding properties because it tends to swell up in tissues.

The first synthetic absorbable suture material was poly-1-lactide but this never gained popularity. Polyglycolic acid (Dexon) was introduced in 1969 and has stood the test of time. It is a polymerised hydroxyacetic acid which is liquified and formed into filaments. These are stretched and braided. Different thicknesses are produced by varying the number of filaments. This material has low tissue reactivity and is absorbed in 60–90 days by slow hydrolysis. Its main problem, high tissue drag, has been largely solved by coating with silicone (Dexon-S).

Polydioxane (PDS) has recently been introduced. It is a polymer of para-dioxanone which is melted and extended into monofilament fibres. These fibres are then orientated and heat set. This material is flexible, with little tissue drag and good knot-tying characteristics, and retains its strength for a long time.

Silk is the oldest non-absorbable suture in use and was made popular by Kocher and Halsted, who became dissatisfied with catgut. Silk is produced from the silkworm larva thread, which consists mainly of protein. The fibre is braided to produce better handling and strength. Floss silk was loosely twisted and is no longer used. Silk is stronger than catgut and can be boiled or autoclaved. Because it tends to absorb fluid it is treated with silicone or wax to render it non-permeable. Although tissue drag is reduced, this unfortunately makes knots less secure.

Cotton is rarely used. It is produced from the long fibre of Egyptian cotton, which is spun. It produces vigorous tissue reaction, like silk, and has poor tensile strength.

Linen is made from twisted staple flax fibres. It is stronger than cotton, produces vigorous tissue reaction, handles well and is cheap.

Synthetic non-absorbable sutures are exemplified by nylon, a synthetic polyamide which is produced as mono or multifilament. Although nylon is strong it loses its strength after six months in tissues and has poor knot-tying qualities, especially in its monofilament form. It is also brittle and tends to snap.

Newer synthetic materials are made of polyesters, polyethylenes or polypropylene. They are also non-reactive, and have better tensile strength and knot-tying qualities.

Stainless steel suture was popularised by Babcock but is now rarely used except, perhaps, in tendon repairs and closure of sternotomy. It is available as monofilament or multifilament. In spite of its strength it eventually undergoes metal fatigue and fragments. Although knots are secure it tends to break if kinked. The ends should be buried because they are liable to produce sinuses and local pain.

Suture material sizes are the source of considerable confusion. Metric numbers refer to the diameter of suture in tenths of a millimetre. The old gauge system was based on the non-absorbable suture diameter in inches. These figures do not apply to non-boilable catgut because it becomes swollen in the packaging fluid and it is therefore one size bigger than the non-absorbable suture of the same gauge (4.0 catgut equals 3.0 silk).

Forrester, J.C. (1972) Suture materials and their use. *British Journal of Hospital Medicine*, November 1972, 578-592.

Ferguson, J.H.L. (1956) Ligature and suture materials. In *Operative Surgery* (ed. Rob, C. and Smith, R.), Vol. I, pp. 5-8. Butterworth, London.

Morgan, M.N. (1969) New synthetic absorbable suture material. *British Medical Journal*, 1969, **2**, 308

Chusak, R.B. and Dibbell, D.G. (1983) Clinical experience with polydioxanone monofilament absorbable sutures in plastic surgery. *Plastic and Reconstructive Surgery*, **72**, 217-220.

Babcock, W.W. (1947) *Surgical Clinics of North America*, **27**, 1435

7.3 Surgical gloves

Most surgeons use gloves during surgical or therapeutic procedures as a matter of course. Their introduction into surgical practice was one of the most important milestones in surgery. They are an essential barrier between patient and surgeon, serving to protect both from infection.

Although William Halsted is often credited with the introduction of rubber surgical gloves into practice it is certain that gloves were being used as early as the 1850s. From the evidence available it appears that Halsted in fact rarely wore gloves during surgery. The early surgical gloves were made of thick vulcanised rubber. They were reusable and after use were washed, repaired and sterilised.

The present day surgical gloves are made from latex rubber. Porcelain formers in the shape of hands of various sizes are dipped into latex solution and when removed are coated by a thin layer of latex. By passing the coated porcelain formers through ovens the latex is vulcanised and after a period of cooling the gloves are peeled off.

In order to produce an outer textured and inner smooth surface the gloves are manufactured inside out. To prevent the dry surface of gloves sticking together they must be dusted with a powder. Gloves are supplied with a sachet of powder to facilitate donning. The use of powder in the manufacture of gloves and for donning has recently stimulated a lot of interest. Currently, starch powder is used, but lycopodium spores and talc were in use prior to its introduction. There is both clinical and experimental evidence that starch powder can lead to 'starch peritonitis' and some post-operative adhesions. Starch peritonitis is probably due to a specific hypersensitivity to this material. Starch powder can be removed by scrubbing gloved hands with providone iodine surgical scrub (Betadine) for one minute, followed by scrubbing with sterile water for 30 seconds. This procedure is almost 100% effective in removing starch granules from the glove surface.

Recently LRC Products Ltd have developed a new glove which is coated on the inside with a hydrogel polymer. Preliminary animal experiments have shown that this material produces fewer adhesions than the standard surgical glove.

Miller, J.M. (1982) William Stewart Halsted and the use of surgical rubber glove. *Surgery*, **92**, 541-543

Halsted, W.S. (1913) Ligature and suture material. The employment of fine silk in preference to catgut and the advantages of transfixion of tissue and vessels in control of haemorrhage. *Journal of the American Medical Association*, **60**, 1119

Mitchell, J.M. (1945) The introduction of rubber gloves for use in surgical operations. *Annals of Surgery*, **122**, 905.

Randers-Pehron, J. (1960) *The Surgeon's Glove*. Charles C. Thomas, Springfield, Illinois.

Jagelman, D.G. and Ellis, H. (1973) Starch and intraperitoneal adhesion formation *British Journal of Surgery*, **60**, 111-114

Lennox, M. (1983) Studies on starch free gloves. In: *Intestinal Adhesions: The Problem* (ed. Ellis, H. and Lennox, M.). LRC Products Ltd, London.

7.4 Implants

The ideal implant should mimic the tissues or organ it is designed to replace, whether in its size, shape or consistency. It should be permanently tolerated by the host's tissues and should not predispose to infection. The tissue response should not alter its characteristics and the material should not be carcinogenic.

Normal wound healing depends on clotting, replacement of the clot by granulation tissue, scar formation and epithelialisation. Any matter present in the wound, whether autogenous or foreign, will interfere with this process of healing. The tissues respond to these foreign bodies by attempting to dissolve them by an enzymatic process, by extrusion to the surface or by formation of a fibrous capsule. Organic materials, such as allografts, are rapidly recognised by the tissues and are promptly rejected. The result is an intense inflammation and the formation of a granuloma. In the presence of infection this process may continue as chronic inflammation. Synthetic materials evoke weaker reaction than allografts. They are usually enclosed by a fibrous capsule which forms a barrier between the tissue and the implant. The presence of bacteria has a profound influence on foreign implants. Although relatively large numbers of bacteria are required to produce wound infection, in the presence of a foreign body the number of bacteria required to establish infection is greatly reduced.

The presence of tissue necrosis and haematoma further increases the possibility of infection by providing a suitable culture medium. Thus the major impediment to successful tissue foreign implant is the body's own defence mechanism.

Sutures are the foreign implant most commonly used in surgery. The basic requirements for sutures are inertness and ability to maintain strength during wound healing. Absorbable sutures are degraded and absorbed. The disadvantages of catgut have led to the introduction of new synthetic absorbable materials. These materials are glycolides or lactides which are degraded by hydrolysis. The tissue reaction is minimal, in comparison to catgut, and their tensile strength is maintained considerably longer. Among the non-absorbable sutures silk still remains popular, mainly because of its superior handling properties. However, when implanted it is degraded to a variable degree and its fragments may act as a nidus for granuloma formation. Tissue and cellular reaction may eventually lead to its extrusion. Synthetic non-absorbable sutures elicit a far weaker tissue reaction and maintain their strength for a long time; of these, polypropylene monofilament is the least reactive and remains in tissues unaltered for many years. Some non-absorbable sutures, especially if braided, are coated to improve their handling properties. Coating materials themselves may increase tissue reaction to these. Stainless steel sutures, although rarely used, produce a variable tissue reaction and are subject to fatigue leading to fragmentation.

Large tissue defects following trauma, resection of tumours, irradiation or sepsis may require reconstruction with the help of implants in the form of a surgical mesh. Metal plates and mesh were used for this purpose after World War II but these were often unsuccessful, resulting in fragmentation and extrusion. Ivalon sponge was the first synthetic material used for this purpose but it was unsatisfactory because of severe fibrosis and unfavourable behaviour in the presence of wound infection. The introduction of polytetrafluoroethylene (Teflon) mesh produced more satisfactory results. Granulation tissue grew through its interstices and, even in the presence of wound infection, the material was not extruded. Its main disadvantage was poor tensile strength resulting in fragmentation. More closely woven Teflon mesh also proved disappointing in the presence of infection because of poor ingrowth of granulation tissue. Polyethylene (Marlex) has a high tensile strength and is very porous, allowing good ingrowth of granulation tissue. It is resistant to fraying and can be cut to required size and shape. However, it can only be resterilised by boiling, because of its low softening and melting point. Polypropylene (Mersilene, Dacron), on the other hand, has a high melting point and can be autoclaved without loss of tensile strength. For that reason it is superior to polyethylene.

Plastic sponges are used in surgery as a means of inducing fibrosis. For example, they are frequently used in rectopexy for rectal prolapse. The initial tissue response to a plastic sponge implant is acute inflammation, followed by invasion by macrophages and the formation of giant cells. The interstices of the sponge are invaded by granulation tissue which, after maturation, results in massive scarring. In plastic and reconstructive surgery the need for soft, pliable, inert materials resulted in the introduction of silicones. These are a group of polymers known as organopoly-siloxanes, consisting of chains of silicon, oxygen and organic radicals. Silastics are rubber compounds formed from silicon by the addition of ferric or aluminim chloride followed by oxidation. Silicones can be manufactured in the form of rubbers, resins, viscous fluids and watery liquids. Silicones are increasingly used for the manufacture of prostheses as well as various forms of catheters. The material is well tolerated by tissues, producing minimal reaction. The early tissue response is mild inflammation, which may subside within six months. The material becomes enveloped by a thin-walled capsule lined by endothelium-like cells, with moderate surrounding fibrosis. There is no significant chronic inflammatory response after six months. There is evidence that silicone fluids are absorbed systemically by phagocytosis and some, as yet unknown, mechanism. There is no evidence of carcinogenesis after long-term implantation.

The expansion of vascular surgery over the last two decades is largely a result of the introduction of synthetic vascular prostheses. These are made of Dacron or Teflon in knitted, woven or velour forms. The inner surface of the graft becomes covered by pseudointima which is composed of a thin layer of fibrin and blood cells. This layer is thrombogenic and if blood flow decreases a thrombus may form resulting in luminal occlusion or embolism. One of the problems with woven or knitted prostheses has been poor anchoring of pseudointima which, if detached, can block off the graft and embolise. Velour prosthesis is porous and contains long loops of yarn arranged perpendicular to the surface. This arrangement allows ingrowth of fibrous tissue which anchors the lining membrane. Because of its porosity the graft may require pre-clotting. These prostheses are suitable for replacement of large vessels but not for smaller vessels because of high incidence of occlusion. Recently a new non-woven polytetrafluoroethylene(PTFE) has been introduced for replacement of smaller vessels and has shown good patency results, comparable to saphenous vein grafts. The material is made in strips which are wound round a mandrel in two layers. This two-layer arrangement reduces the possibility of aneurysm formation. The main advantage of PTFE grafts is their smoothness, although they are more rigid than woven or knitted grafts.

Metal has been used for implants since the end of the nineteenth century in the form of plates and screws in orthopaedic operations. However, these attempts often led to disastrous consequences, frequently resulting in amputation. The reason for these failures was the lack of suitable metals which could be tolerated by the tissues. It was not until the 1930s that metals were reintroduced into surgery, with the discovery of stainless steel and cobalt–chromium alloys. Since World War II metal implants have revolutionised orthopaedic surgery beyond recognition. The main reason for the early failure of metal implants, in spite of asepsis, was corrosion. Corrosion can be defined as loss of one or several components of the metal to the surrounding environment. This loss becomes significant when it continues over a long period of time and may weaken the mechanical integrity of the implant. Moreover, the corrosion products may stimulate tissue reaction, resulting in inflammation. Sometimes this corrosion product may be beneficial, in that when it covers the surface of the implant it may act as a barrier between the metal and surrounding tissues.

The artificial hip joint is perhaps the most frequently used metal implant and also a very successful one. The first artificial hip joint was used in 1891 and was made of ivory. Various materials were been used with little success until 1938, when Smith-Petersen carried out a vitallium cup hip arthroplasty. The first entirely stainless steel prosthesis was used by Wiles in 1938. In 1951 McKee developed bone cement (methyl methacrylate) for fixation of metal prostheses to bone. In 1964 Ring developed a metal-to-metal total hip prosthesis which did not prove to be successful because of wear accelerated by metallic debris. In an attempt to eliminate this problem Charnley used a Teflon socket and metal femoral head. The head was, however, shown to be subject to considerable wear. He therefore replaced the Teflon with a high-density polyethylene and introduced a smaller femoral head to reduce frictional resistance. This combination of vitallium and high-density polyethylene has proved to be the most successful to date.

Silver, I.A. (1980) The physiology of wound healing. In: *Wound Healing and Wound Infection* (ed. Hunt, T.K.). Appleton-Century-Crofts, New York.

Salthouse, T.N. (1980) Biologic response to sutures. *Otolaryngology and Head and Neck Surgery*, **88**(6), 658.

Effler, D.B. (1953) Prevention of chest wall defects: use of tantalum and steel mesh. *Journal of Thoracic Surgery*, **26**, 419.

Dietel, M. and Vasic, V. (1979) A secure method of repair of large ventral hernias with Marlex mesh to eliminate tension. *American Journal of Surgery*, **137**, 276-277.

Charlesworth, D. (1980) Arterial replacements. In: *Recent Advances in Surgery 10* (ed. Selwyn Taylor). Churchill Livingstone, Edinburgh.

Venable, C.S. and Stuck, W.G. (1947) *The Internal Fixation of Fractures*. Charles C. Thomas, Springfield, Illinois.

Charnley, J. (1961) Arthroplasty of the hip, a new operation. *Lancet*, 1961, 1, 1129

Charnley, J. Long-term wear studies of high density polyethylene in total hip replacement. *Journal of Bone and Joint Surgery*, **588**, 390.

Rubin, L.R. (ed.) (1983) *Biomaterials in Reconstructive Surgery*. C.V. Mosby, St. Louis.

Part 3 Operative Instruments

Chapter 8 General and Abdominal Surgery

8.1 Knives, scalpels and bistouries
8.2 Scissors
8.3 Haemostatic forceps
8.4 Tissue-grasping forceps
8.5 Dissecting forceps
8.6 Intestinal clamps
8.7 Dissectors, probes and directors
8.8 Needle holders
8.9 Wound retractors
8.10 Cholecystectomy instruments
8.11 Thyroid instruments

8.1 Knives, scalpels and bistouries

A scalpel is a small knife used in surgical and anatomical operations. In surgical practice the term knife refers to a cutting tool, other than scalpel, and is usually reserved for amputation knives, which are substantially larger than scalpels.

The scalpel is synonymous with surgery. It has been invariably used for incision and sometimes for dissection. Over the centuries the scalpel has developed from a metal blade with a handle of bone, ivory or wood to an all-steel instrument. Today scalpels consist of a metal handle and a disposable stainless steel blade of various shapes and sizes. Amputation knives have been known since before Roman times and although now rarely used, were an important part of the surgeon's armamentarium. Until 1846, when anaesthesia was introduced, amputations were performed on conscious patients and speed was of the essence. Perhaps the most famous surgeon connected with amputation was Robert Liston, who was able to perform an above-knee amputation in 25 seconds. It is said that his zeal to break his own record once resulted in the amputation of one of the patient's testicles as well as two of the assistant's fingers at the same time!

Liston's knives were very long, some up to 14 inches, and either straight or curved. This was because he aimed to cut the skin and muscle in a single circular sweep round the limb.

Syme's amputation knife, designed particularly for amputation of the foot, is smaller but very strong.

The bistoury is a long scalpel made in several forms, straight or curved and sharp-pointed or probe-pointed. Its main feature is a blade of uniform

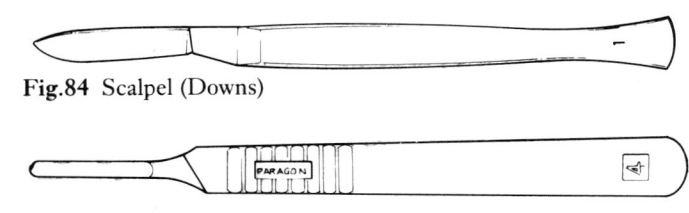

Fig.84 Scalpel (Downs)

Fig.85 Scalpel handle (Downs)

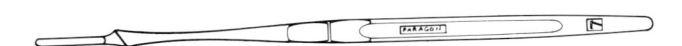

Fig.86 Scalpel handle (Downs)

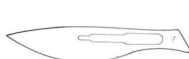

Fig.87 Scalpel blade (Downs)

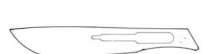

Fig.88 Scalpel blade (Downs)

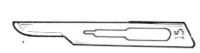

Fig.89 Scalpel blade (Downs)

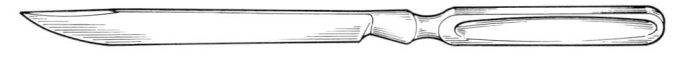

Fig.90 Liston amputation knife (Downs)

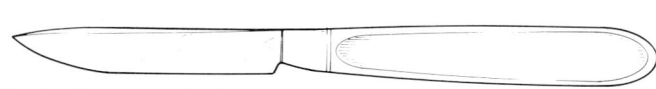

Fig.91 Syme joint knife (Downs)

breadth, with no belly and with a long ventral cutting edge. Fistula bistouries were designed to pass along a fistulous tract and had guarded ends. Cooper's hernia bistoury is a curved bistoury with a blunt end. The blunt end was designed to pass beneath the tight constriction ring of a hernia, followed by the cutting blade which cut the constricting edge without damage to the viscus.

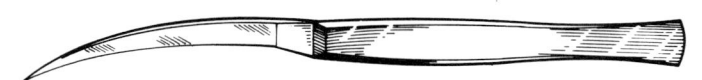

Fig.92 Curved, sharp-pointed bistoury (Downs)

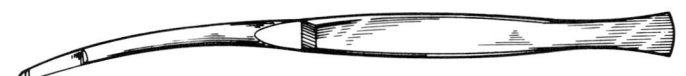

Fig.93 Cooper hernia bistoury (Downs)

8.2 Scissors

Scissors, as we know them today, are of relatively recent design. Before the introduction of the present-day cross-action scissors the instrument was based on a proximal joint with tong-like action. Cutting takes place at the moving point of contact between the edges of the two blades. The angle of the bevel changes according to the material that it must cut. Apart from those used for dressing and stitching most surgical scissors are dissecting scissors and have chamfered ends. On the whole there is no place for sharp-pointed scissors in surgery.

The choice of surgical scissors is vast. They can be long or short, strong or fine, blunt or sharp-pointed, straight or curved either on the flat side or on the edge. More expensive scissors have tungsten-edges which are sharp, tough and long-lasting.

The choice will depend on many factors, and the surgeon's preference is perhaps the most important of these. For surface cutting, short scissors are appropriate, and long scissors are used in deep dissection as in thoracic and pelvic surgery. Curved scissors are more popular for dissection because, with the convexity of blades pointing away from the surgeon, structures being cut on both sides of the tip are visible. It should be realised that the longer the instrument, the more pronounced is the tremor transmitted. Most popular versatile short scissors are Mayo's. They were popularised by the Mayo brothers at the Mayo Clinic, and are supplied straight or curved for fine surgical dissection.

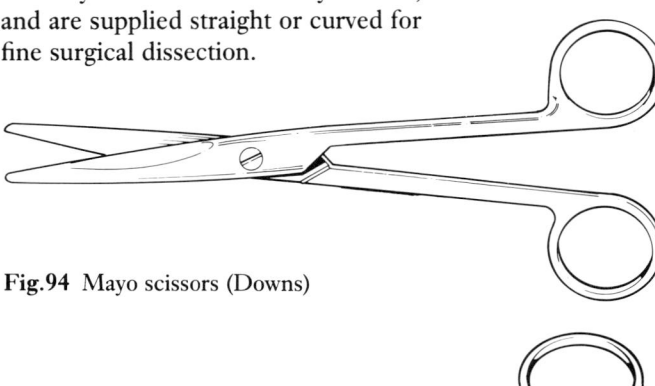

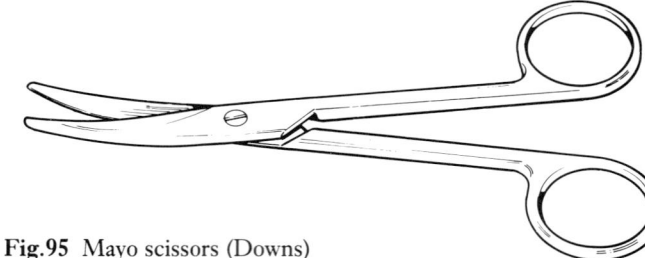

Fig.94 Mayo scissors (Downs)

Fig.95 Mayo scissors (Downs)

The most popular intermediate-length scissors are McInde's, which are curved and 7 inches long. They are, however, quite delicate and easily damaged if used inappropriately.

For deeper dissection and cutting, long scissors (9–11 inches) are required because the operator's hand is then out of the way and because small instruments are easily left behind in the body cavities. The choice lies between Nelson's and Metzenbaum's. Metzenbaum's scissors, although slightly longer (9.5 inches), have shorter and thinner blades and should be used for finer dissection. Nelson's scissors (9 inches long), originally designed for thoracic surgery, are stronger and better all-rounders.

In pelvic surgery, division of tough ligaments and pedicles requires strong scissors with blunt edges. Lloyd Davies's are typical of such scissors. Abel's scissors are perhaps an exaggerated example of this requirement.

8.3 Haemostatic forceps

The function of haemostatic forceps is to stop or prevent bleeding. They look very much like scissors and incorporate a rachet lock on springy steel handles and crushing jaws instead of blades. The handles end in rings to accommodate the fingers. The tissue is grasped between the jaw tips.

Before the nineteenth century haemostasis was achieved by cautery or by using ordinary tissue forceps with a ring on the outside to maintain

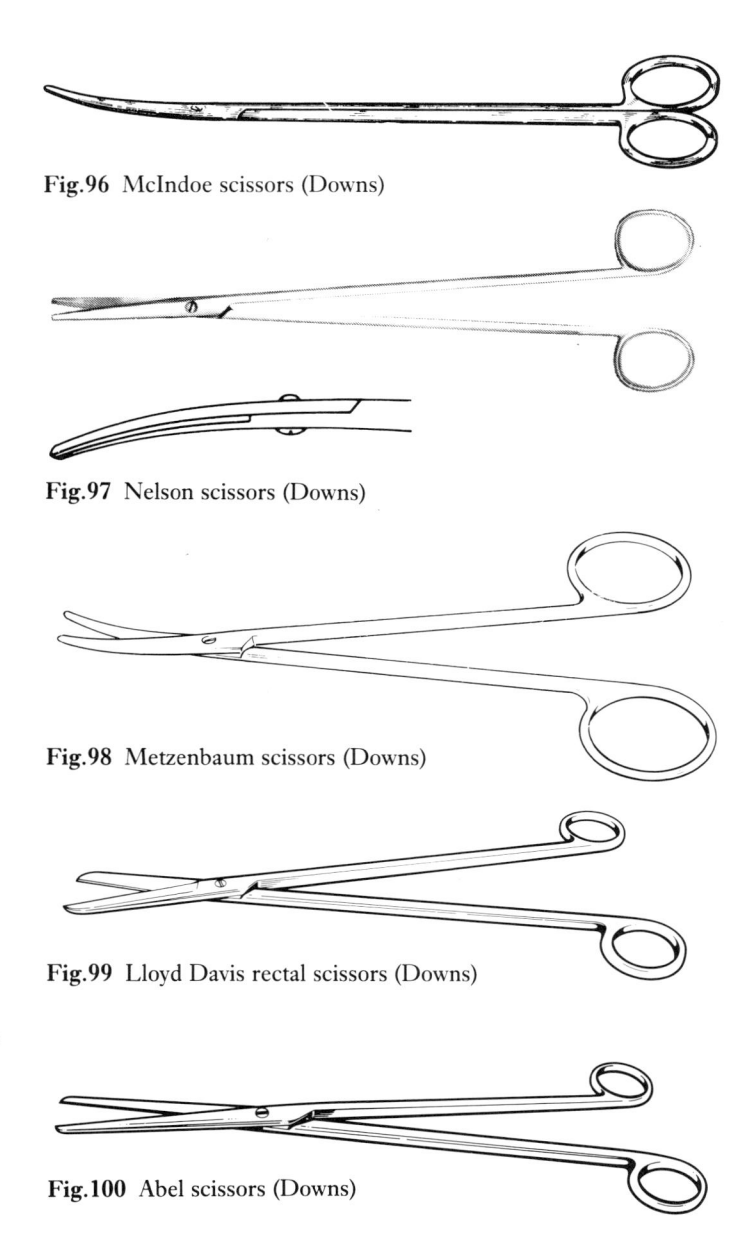

Fig.96 McIndoe scissors (Downs)

Fig.97 Nelson scissors (Downs)

Fig.98 Metzenbaum scissors (Downs)

Fig.99 Lloyd Davis rectal scissors (Downs)

Fig.100 Abel scissors (Downs)

occlusion of the jaws. At the beginning of the nineteenth century, torsion of arteries became fashionable as a means of haemostasis. In 1840 Charriere produced new spring forceps with crossed jaws. These are now known as Dieffenbach's artery forceps.

The first artery forceps, as we know them today, were designed by Pean, followed by Spencer Wells and Ochsner. Who was the first still remains in dispute. Artery forceps are connected with the names of famous surgeons of the late nineteenth and early twentieth centuries: Doyen, Kocher, Halsted, Cushing, Crile and others.

They can be classified on the basis of the design of the jaws. Fine and strong, short and long, curved and straight. The opposing surfaces of jaws can have longitudinal, transverse or oblique serrations. Some, such as Kocher's, have interdigitating teeth at the tip.

The joints may be simple or of the box-lock type, in which one blade passes through a channel in the other blade. The ring handles allow pressure to be exerted in all directions, resulting in opening or closing of the jaws.

Fig.101 Spencer Wells artery forceps (Downs)

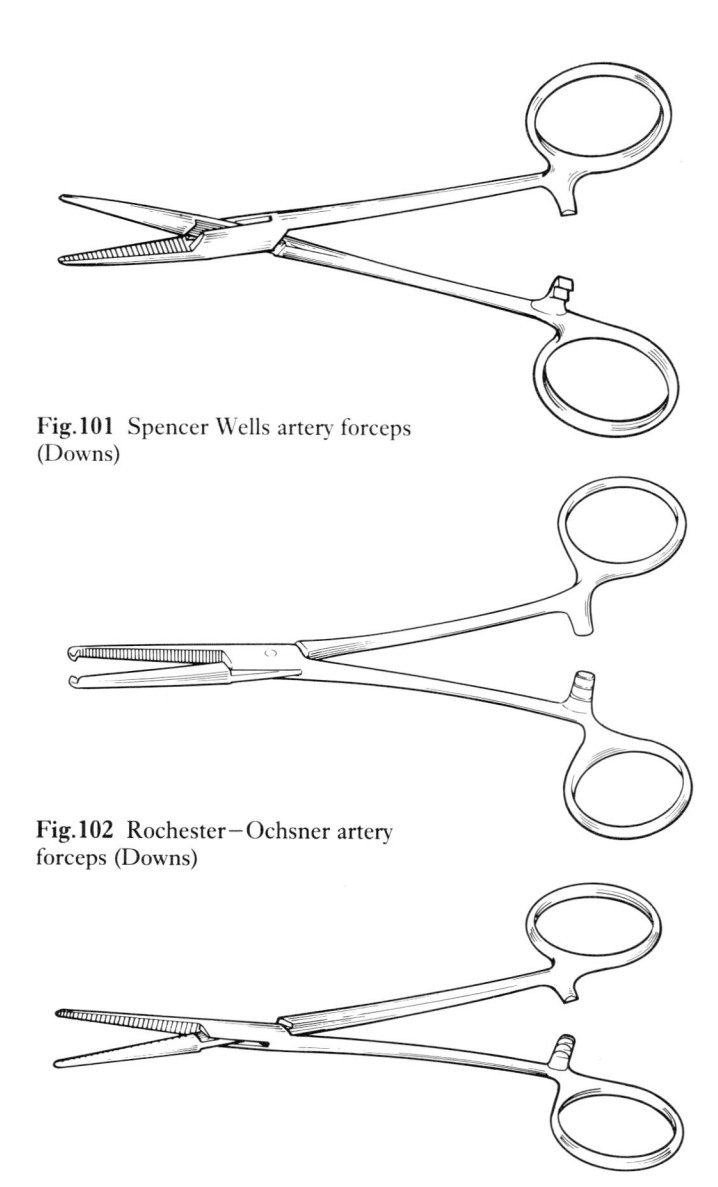

Fig.102 Rochester–Ochsner artery forceps (Downs)

Fig.103 Crile artery forceps (Downs)

8.4 Tissue-grasping forceps

Tissue-grasping forceps are designed to grasp tissues without crushing them so as to allow their manipulation. They resemble haemostatic forceps except that the blades approximate only at the tips. The tips are usually made in the

GENERAL AND ABDOMINAL SURGERY 87

Fig.104 Cushing artery forceps (Downs)

Fig.105 Dunhill artery forceps (Downs)

Fig.106 Moynihan artery forceps (Downs)

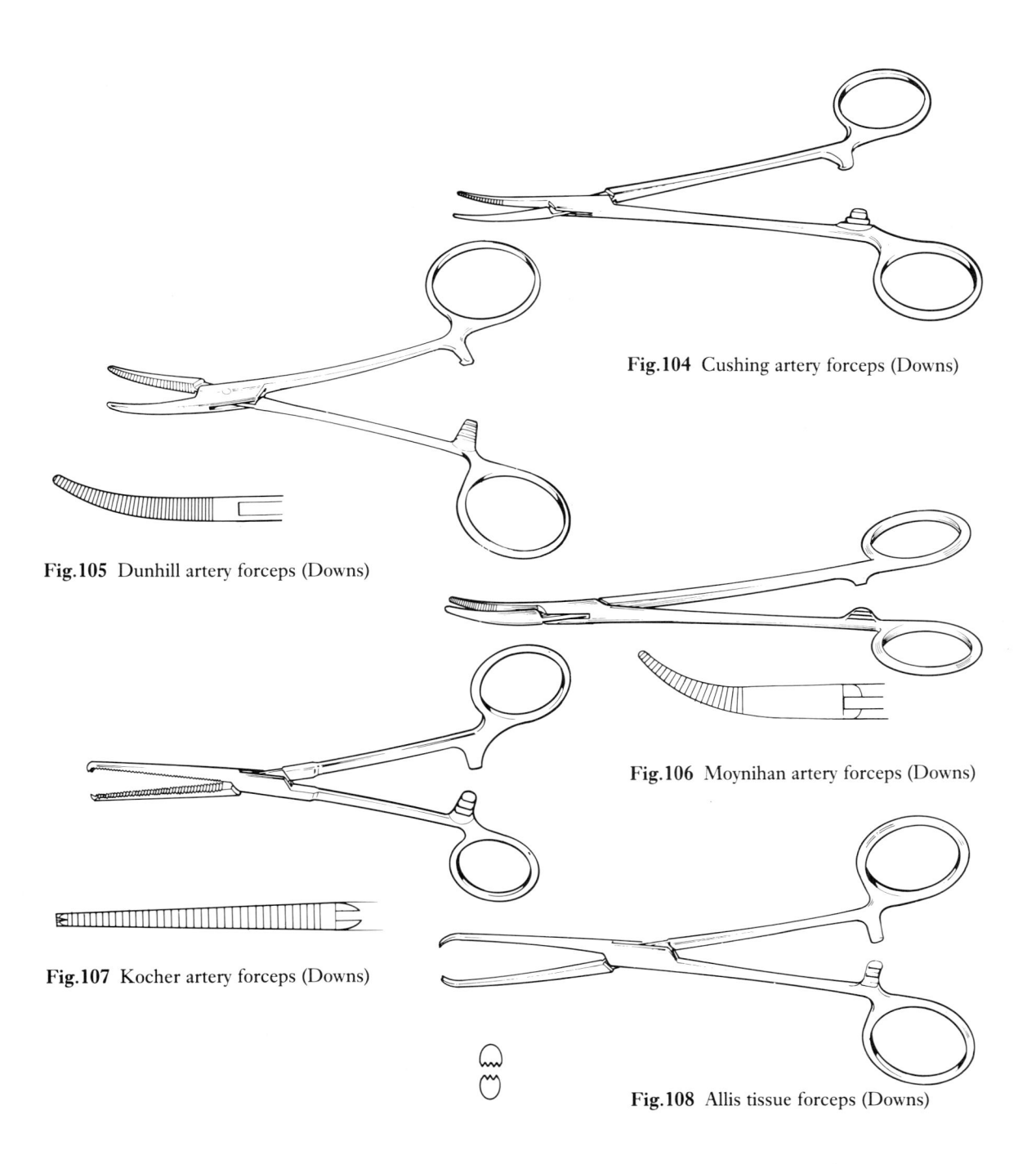

Fig.107 Kocher artery forceps (Downs)

Fig.108 Allis tissue forceps (Downs)

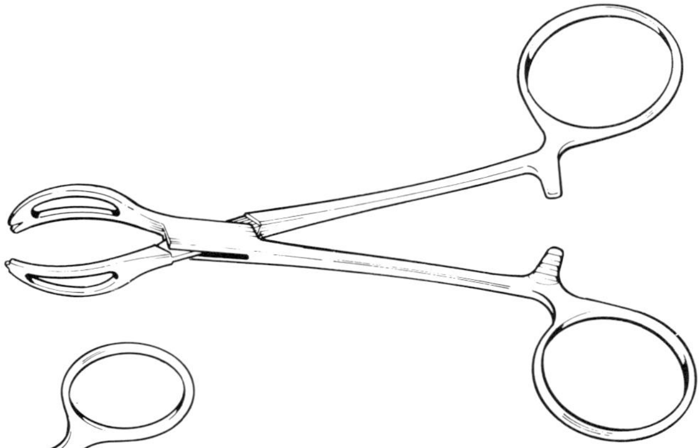

88 OPERATIVE INSTRUMENTS

Fig.109 Lane tissue forceps (Downs)

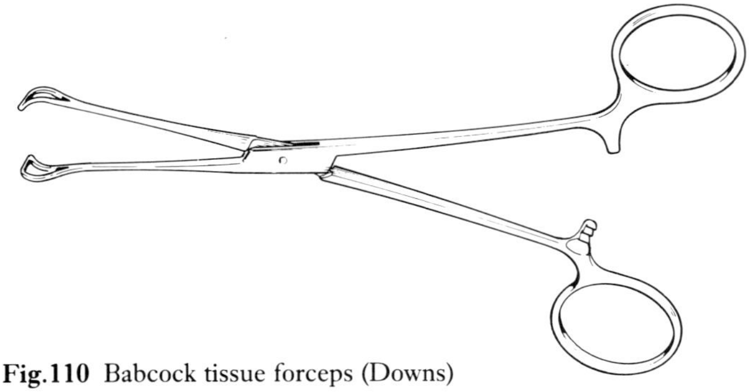

Fig.110 Babcock tissue forceps (Downs)

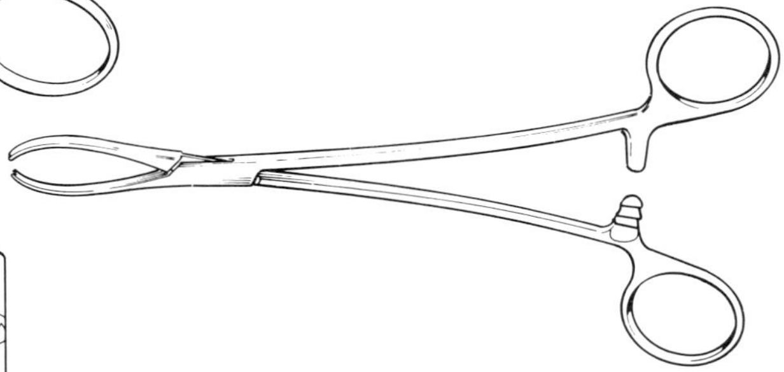

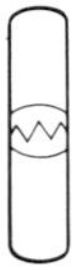

Fig.111 Littlewood tissue forceps (Downs)

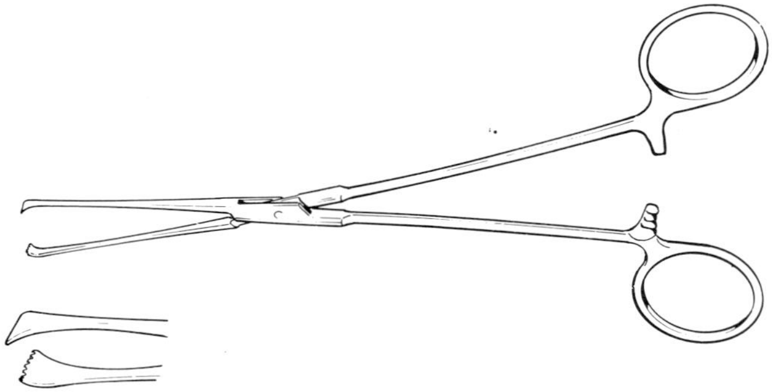

Fig.112 Stile tissue forceps (Downs)

form of teeth to reduce tissue damage and improve grip.

Most commonly used tissue forceps are Babcock's, Allis's, Duval's and Lane's.

8.5 Dissecting forceps

These are also called thumb forceps because their shafts are closed by the surgeon's thumb. They are used to grasp tissue in order to facilitate dissection or suturing, and are divided into toothed and non-toothed varieties.

Teeth can be single or multiple or arranged in longitudinal rows as in modern vascular-tissue forceps. Toothed forceps give a better grip on tissue but they are also more traumatic. The least traumatic are forceps of the non-toothed variety with fine transverse serrations, or those of the cardiovascular pattern with longitudinal fine-toothed serrations.

8.6 Intestinal clamps

Intestinal clamps are large self-retaining forceps with a primary function to occlude the bowel lumen. The reason for using intestinal clamps is threefold; they occlude the viscus lumen and prevent spillage of infected bowel contents, temporarily occlude circulation in the bowel wall and thus keep the operative field free of blood and, finally, facilitate anastomosis by allowing the bowel ends to be approximated and manipulated. Bowel clamps are non-crushing or crushing.

Non-crushing clamps serve to

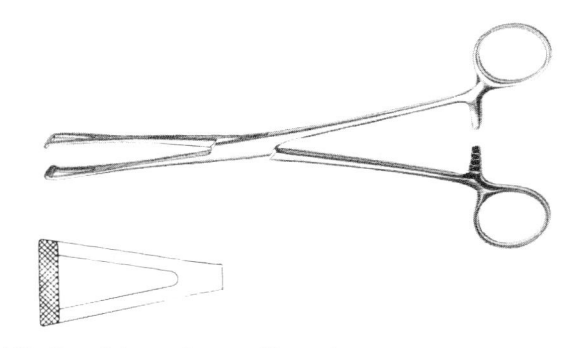

Fig.113 Duval tissue forceps (Downs)

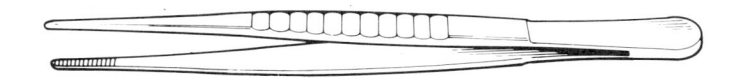

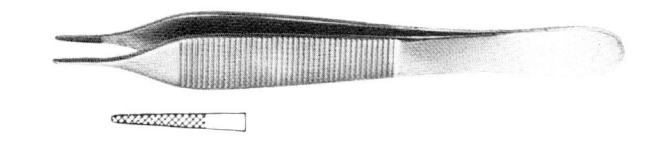

Fig.114 Canadian dissecting forceps (Downs)

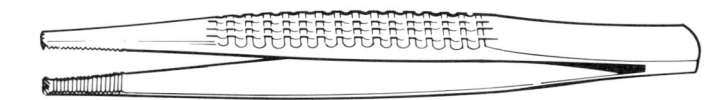

Fig.115 Mitchell dissecting forceps (Downs)

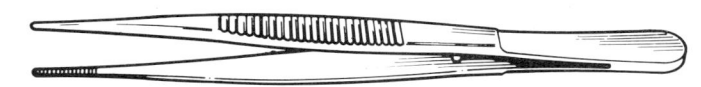

Fig.116 Mitchell dissecting forceps (Downs)

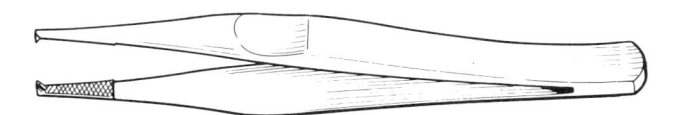

Fig.117 Lane dissecting forceps (Downs)

Fig.118 Adson dissecting forceps (Downs)

occlude temporarily the bowel lumen without permanent damage to the blood supply. Some may also have haemostatic action, which is particularly important in gastric and proximal small-bowel surgery.

The simplest non-crushing intestinal clamp is exemplified by Doyen's. This instrument, first demonstrated in 1887, has long straight or curved jaws. The jaws have longitudinal fine serrations and are elastic. When closed, the slightly bowed jaws meet at the tips and approach each other in the centre as the rachet is tightened. This action ensures that the bowel is subjected to the minimum of pressure without slipping.

Because the highest pressure is exerted at the tips, these should therefore be free of the bowel wall to prevent irreversible damage to the blood supply.

The Kocher soft stomach clamp is of similar design but in addition has a metal rocking piece at the tips which holds them together and prevents the bowel from slipping.

The Eve non-crushing intestinal forceps have transverse serrations and longitudinal fenestrations along the length of both jaws. This design has no advantage over the longitudinal striations of the Doyen clamp. The Arbuthnot Lane twin intestinal clamp is still popular and consists of two non-crushing clamps, which can be joined together by a screw joint proximally and a fixed square ring on the tip of one of the clamp into which the

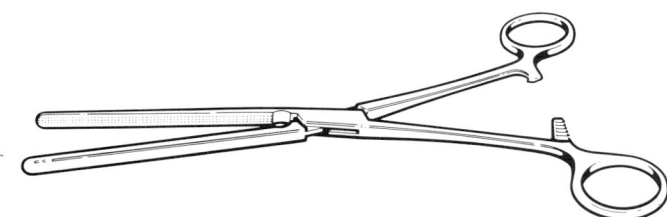

Fig.119 Doyen intestinal clamp (Downs)

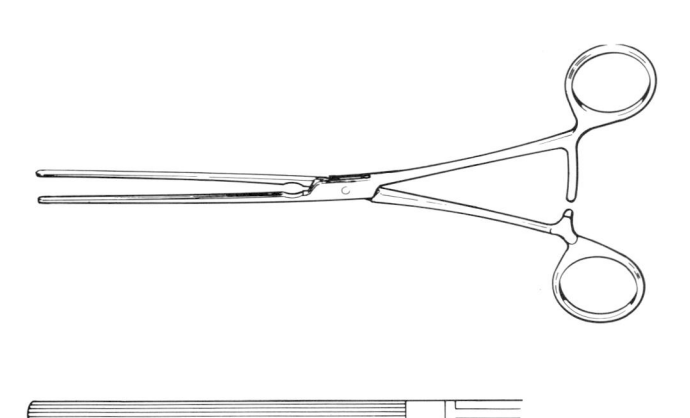

Fig.120 Kocher intestinal clamp (Downs)

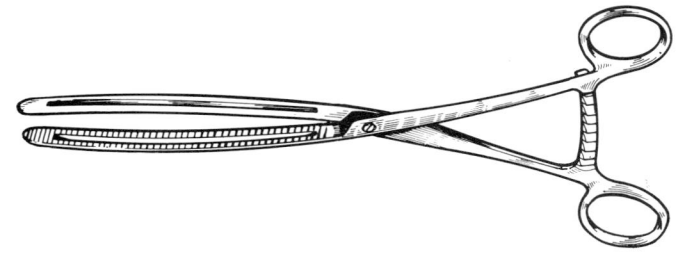

Fig.121 Eve intestinal forceps (Downs)

opposite clamp is slotted. This instrument and its many modifications, such as the Abadie twin clamp, were designed specifically for gastroenterostomy. One of the clamps

GENERAL AND ABDOMINAL SURGERY 91

is applied across the stomach, or part of its wall, and the other over a loop of the jejunum. The clamps are then occluded and joined by the ring and screw joint mechanism.

Clamps, for rectal occlusion, such as Lloyd-Davies's have suitably angled jaws, usually at 75 – 90°. Sometimes rubber tubing is inserted over the jaws in the hope that this will lessen damage to the bowel blood supply. In fact, the opposite is true because the tubing reduces the space between the blades and, moreover, the clamp has a greater tendency to slip off.

Crushing intestinal clamps not only close the bowel lumen but also crush and devitalise a narrow segment of the bowel wall. The crushed segment has to be excised after clamp removal if an end-to-end anastomosis is carried out. If used to occlude a lumen which will subsequently be closed, as the duodenum in Polya gastrectomy, the crushed segment can be left intact and simply inverted.

The Payr clamp is the most popular of crushing clamps. It is a lever-action clamp, with four joints. The proximal joints operate the distal joint and when the jaws are occluded further approximation of the handles results in firm closure without the tendency for the handles to spring apart. The jaws have longitudinal serrations.

Other crushing clamps are of the forceps and ratchet design with robust non-elastic jaws. These are typified by the Lang Stevenson intestinal clamp. Some have additional interlocking teeth at the tips to prevent the

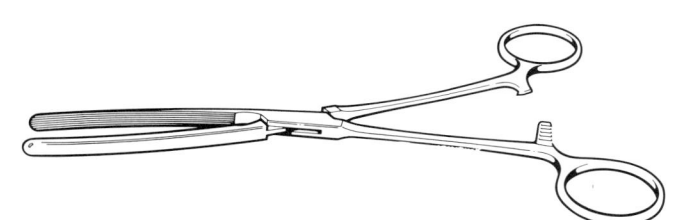

Fig.122 Lane intestinal clamp (Downs)

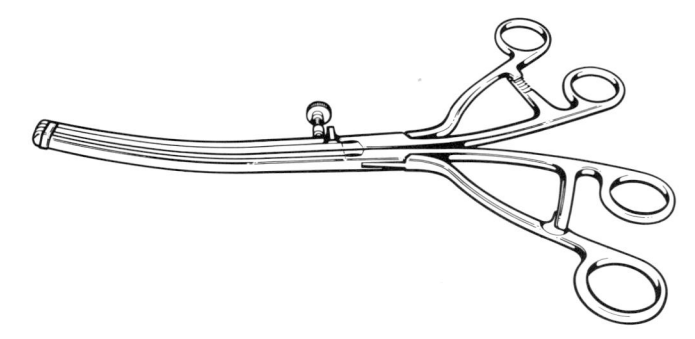

Fig.123 Lane twin anastomotic clamp (Downs)

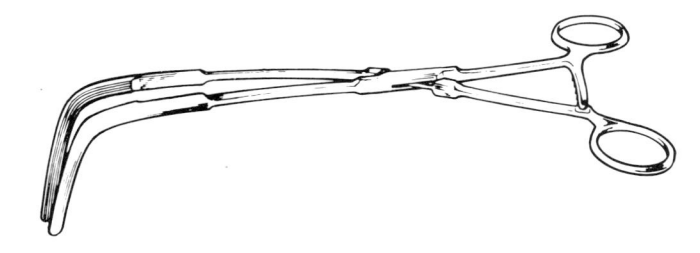

Fig.124 Lloyd Davies rectal occlusion forceps (Downs)

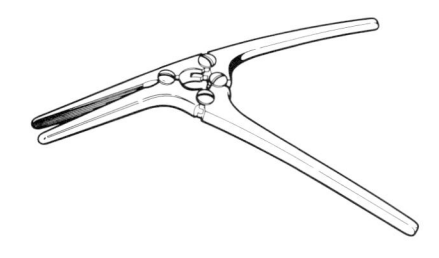

Fig.125 Payr intestinal clamp (Downs)

instrument from slipping.

The de Martel crushing clamp is used mainly in surgery of the large bowel. It consists of three small, straight clamps which are applied in parallel by means of closing forceps. Before the forceps are removed the clamps are secured by means of hinged locks. The middle clamp is then unlocked and removed and the bowel divided between the two remaining lateral clamps.

The Zachary Cope modification of de Martel's clamp is more popular as the three clamps are loaded into a lever-action closing device before application and this makes occlusion easier to carry out. As in the de Martel, the catch locks are applied or disengaged with a tommy bar.

The advantage of these clamps is that they are very small and their firm crushing action makes soiling unlikely. They are also useful in the formation of an end colostomy as, owing to their small size, they can be passed through the abdominal opening without hindrance.

8.7 Dissectors, probes and directors

A dissector is any instrument used for blunt separation of tissues, whether it be the point of a pair of scissors, a haemostat or dissecting forceps. However, there are some instruments designed specifically as tissue dissectors. The MacDonald–Stiles aneurysm needle and dissector is two-ended, one end being straight and the

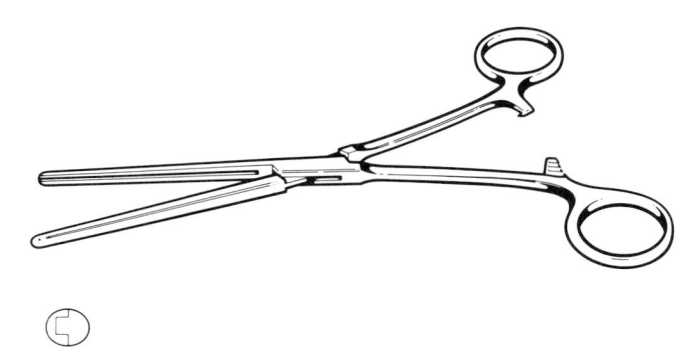

Fig.126 Lang Stevenson intestinal clamp (Downs)

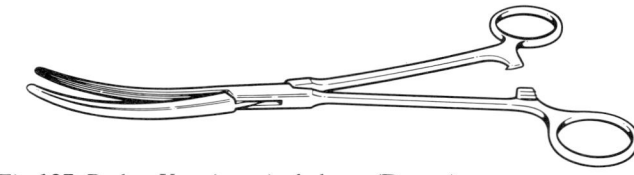

Fig.127 Parker Kerr intestinal clamp (Downs)

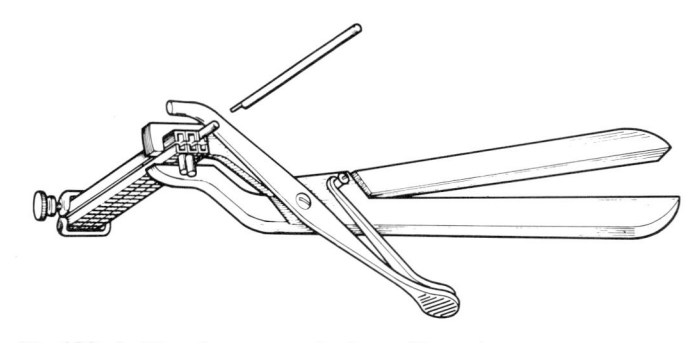

Fig.128 de Martel anastomosis clamp (Downs)

other curved. The curved end serves to pass under a vessel in the same way as an aneurysm needle, and a ligature is passed through a small hole at the tip of the curved blade. Without the hole the instrument is called plain MacDonald.

The Watson Cheyne double-ended dissector is used for dissection of vessels, nerves and glands. One end is in the shape of a fine probe, and the other is curved and flattened. Kocher's thyroid dissector, now used almost exclusively for isolation of superior thyroid pedicle, was originally designed as a universal dissector.

Probes are usually used for investigating sinuses or fistulas and for detection of their depth. They may be soft and malleable or rigid, curved or straight, wide or narrow.

Brodie's fistula probe-director is best known because its flat expanded end has a frenulum split which was used to protect the tongue during frenuloplasty for tongue-tie.

Directors are narrow blunt-ended instruments with a groove along which a bistoury may be passed. They were used for laying open sinuses or fistulas and also in cases of strangulated hernias.

8.8 Needle holders

Initially it should be mentioned that many types of needle can be held between the fingers. Needle holders are modified box-lock forceps designed to hold curved needles. The surgeon should thus be able to manipulate the needle with ease during suturing. Since needle holders are designed to hold needles it is important, when choosing one, to bear that fact in mind. Fine needle holders are damaged by large needles and small needles are damaged by large needle holders.

For suturing skin a short needle

Fig.129 Zachary Cope modification of de Martel clamp (Downs)

Fig.130 Mikulicz enterostomy clamp (Downs)

Fig.131 MacDonald dissector (Downs)

Fig.132 Watson Cheyne dissector (Downs)

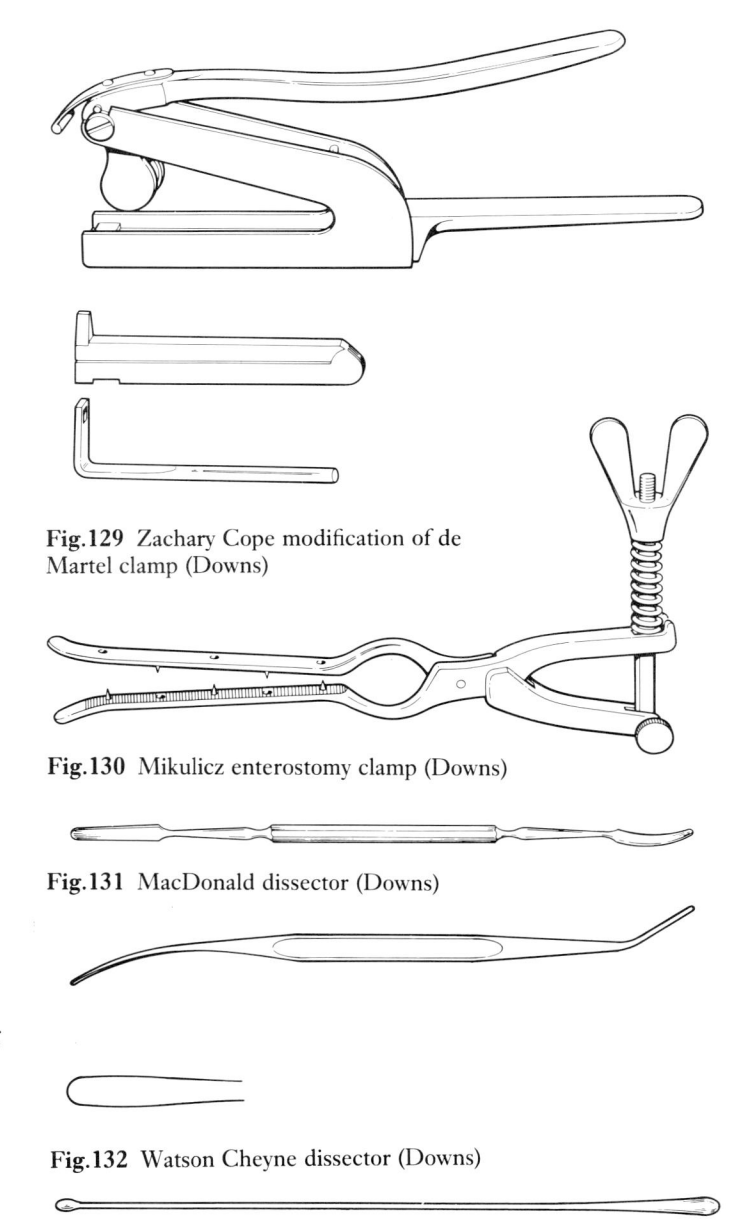

Fig.133 Sinus probe (Downs)

holder is best, such as Mayo's, and for finer needles Gillie's is the most efficient. For work in deep cavities the handles need to be long. There is little use for complex needle holders such as Halsted's. This beautiful instrument easily gets damaged and if not well balanced can become a source of annoyance.

For suturing in deep cavities such as the pelvis, the Naunton Morgan needle holder can be used to advantage. Because it utilises two joints the space occupied by the handles is thus reduced. This needle holder has disadvantages during instrument knot-tying, as suture material can easily get caught in some of the joint projections.

Tungsten-carbide jaws prolong the life of the instrument considerably and are less likely to result in the needle slipping or turning. Reverdin's needle is in fact needle and holder in one. The needle is fixed to the handle and the needle's eye can be opened by a spring shutter which is activated by squeezing the handles together. The suture material is hooked over the eye, the handle is released and the needle withdrawn, pulling the suture behind with it.

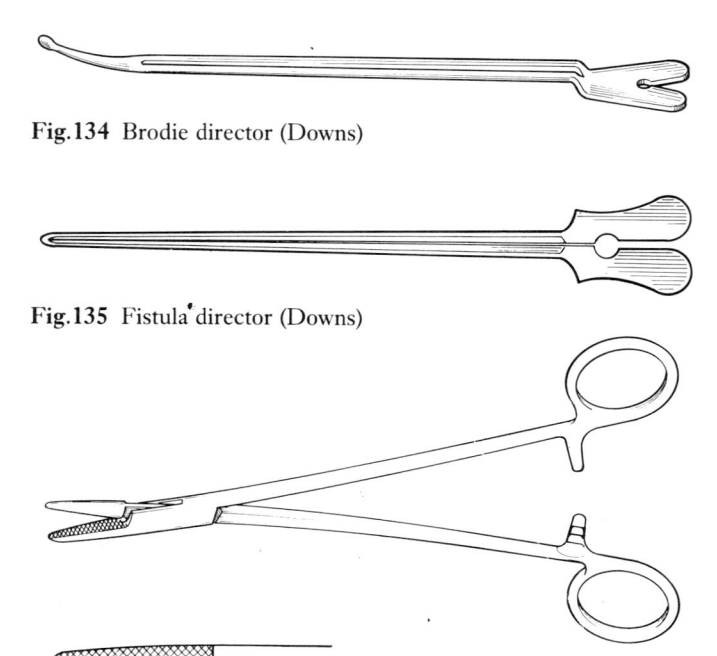

Fig.134 Brodie director (Downs)

Fig.135 Fistula director (Downs)

Fig.136 Mayo needle holder (Downs)

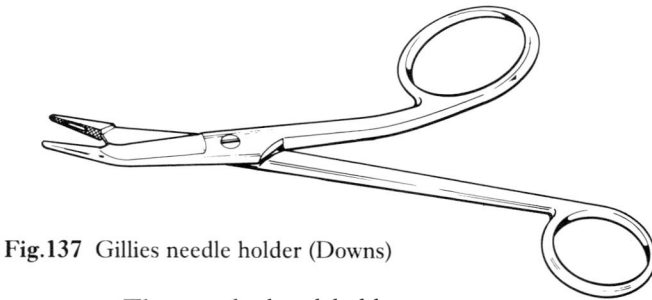

Fig.137 Gillies needle holder (Downs)

8.9 Wound retractors

Good exposure is one of the requisites of successful surgery. Retraction of the wound can be achieved by using the assistant's hand or tissue-grasping forceps applied to the wound edge.

Instruments designed specifically to improve exposure are called wound retractors. They can be hand-held or self-retaining.

Hand-held retractors have a handle and a retracting blade. The Langenbeck wound retractor is the most popular of the small hand-held retractors and demonstrates their basic design. It has a ring-shaped handle with serrations, and long shaft with a right-angled retracting narrow blade. The short length of the retracting blade makes it suitable for superficial retraction only.

Other small retractors differ in the shape of the retracting blade, which may be hook-shaped or curved. Larger retractors are intended to retract a wider area and to expose deeper structures.

The Morris retractor is essentially a large Langenbeck retractor with a wider and longer retracting blade. It is useful for retraction of abdominal wounds. It was originally designed as a kidney retractor.

The Kelly retractor is recognisable by its 19 cm long and gently curved blade. It is particularly suitable for cholecystectomy.

Deaver's retractor, although commonly used, is not popular with surgeon's assistants. It is made of a flat piece of stainless steel with a flat handle, without serrations and of the same width as the curved retracting blade. The handle is uncomfortable if gripped for long periods. The upcurved end of the handle is designed to prevent the assistant's hand from slipping. This instrument is made in several sizes and is therefore a good general-purpose retractor.

Some hand-held retractors were developed for a specific purpose.

The Lloyd-Davies retractor, for example, was designed for deep retraction in rectal surgery. The long blade is concave in cross-section and

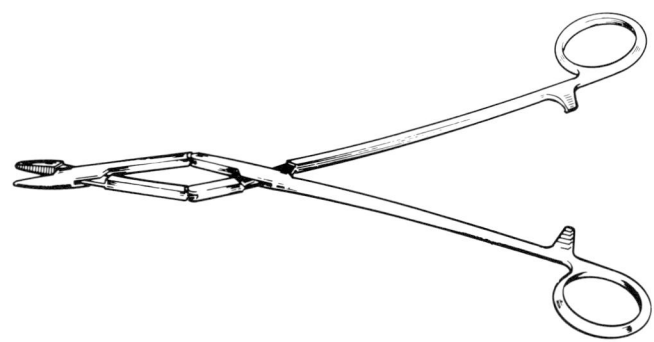

Fig.138 Naunton Morgan needleholder (Downs)

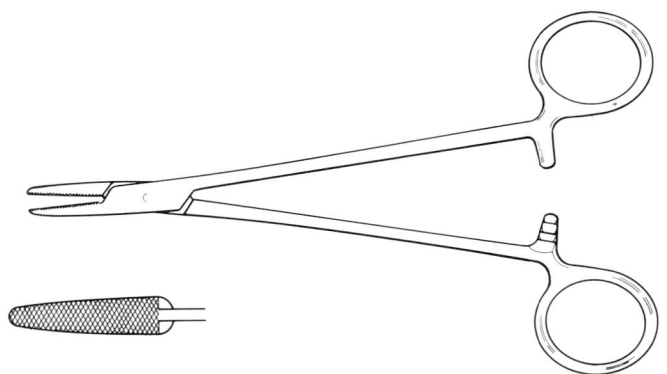

Fig.139 Mayo-Hegar needleholder (Downs)

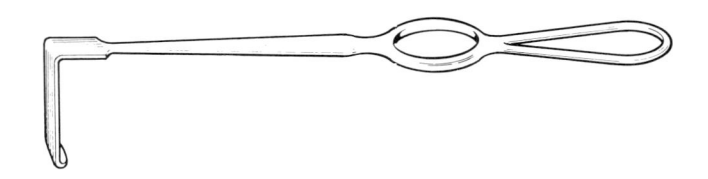

Fig.140 Langenbeck retractor (Downs)

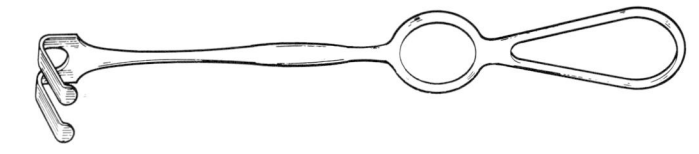

Fig.141 Ollier retractor (Downs)

its end may be tapered. A narrow, incurved lip at the end facilitates exposure in low anterior resection of the rectum by retracting the bladder neck or prostate.

Self-retaining retractors obviate the need for continuous wound retraction by the assistant. Small self-retaining retractors are typified by Travers's retractor, which consists of two retractors connected by a screw joint. The handles have finger rings at the end and occlusion of these separates the right-angled jaws. The retraction is maintained by a cam ratchet. Large abdominal wound retractors can be of similar design, although they are more robust.

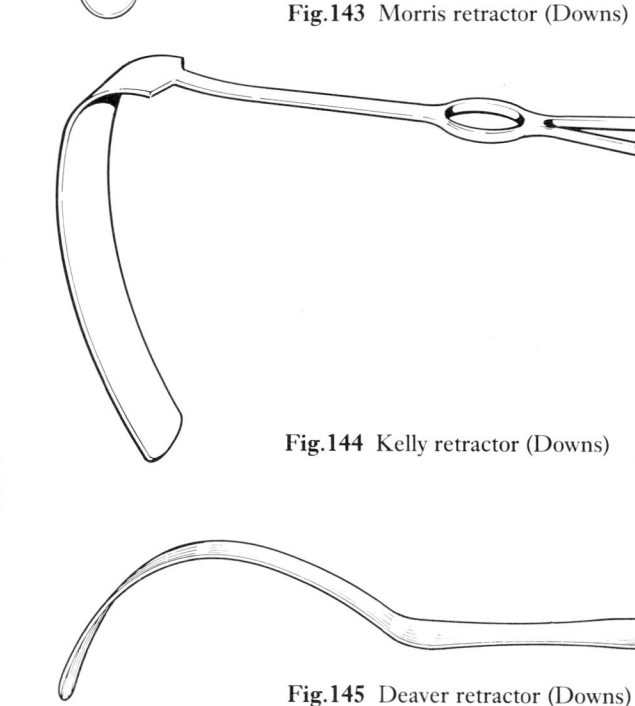

Fig.143 Morris retractor (Downs)

Fig.144 Kelly retractor (Downs)

Fig.142 Czerny retractor (Downs)

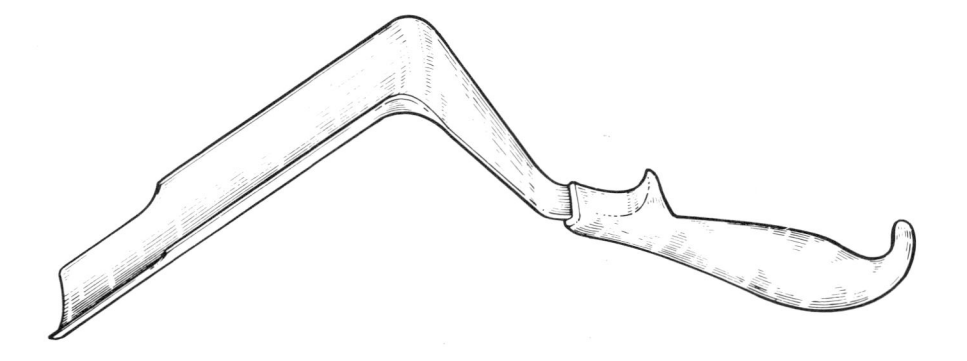

Fig.145 Deaver retractor (Downs)

Fig.146 Lloyd Davies retractor (Downs)

GENERAL AND ABDOMINAL SURGERY 97

Balfour or similar retractors employ a transverse bar to which one blade is fixed, the other moving along it to provide lateral traction. Alternatively, this lateral retraction is achieved by a locking key and rack, as in some thoracic retractors. The transverse bar may be used to add a third retractor at right angles to the other two. This blade is particularly suitable for retraction of the lower part of the wound in pelvic surgery.

The Dennis Browne retractor consists of a circular frame and four or more separate blades. The lower

Fig.147 Travers retractor (Downs)

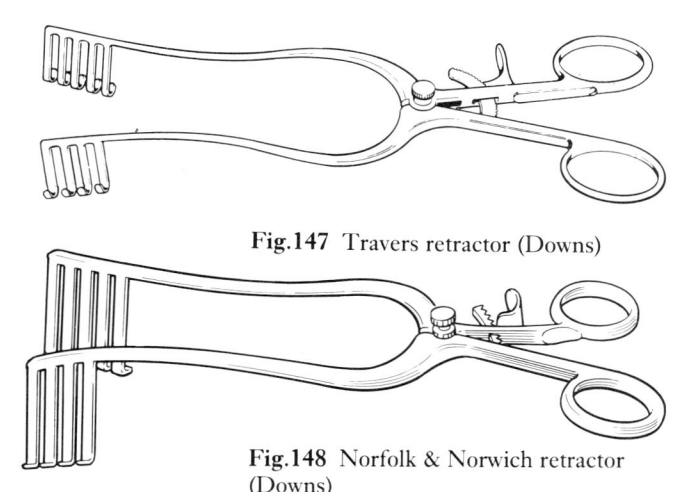

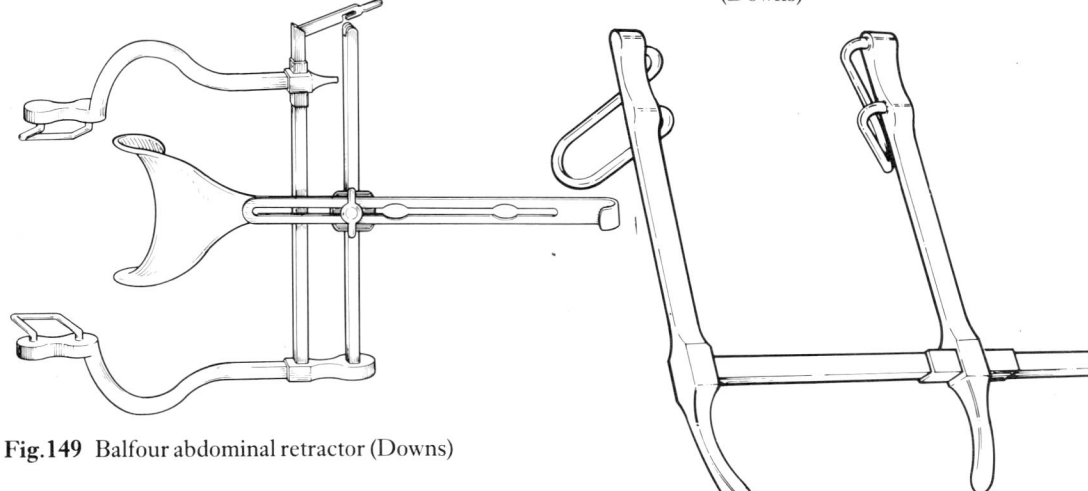

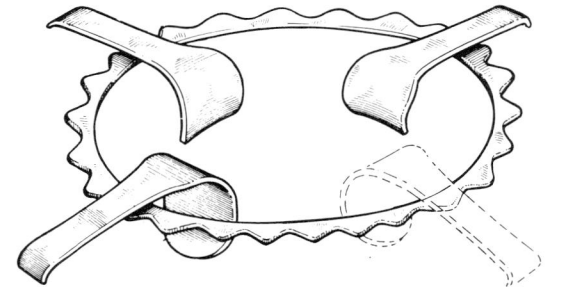

Fig.148 Norfolk & Norwich retractor (Downs)

Fig.149 Balfour abdominal retractor (Downs)

Fig.150 Gosset retractor (Downs)

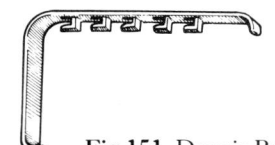

Fig.151 Dennis Browne retractor (Downs)

surface of the shaft of each blade is provided with a number of right-angled hooks which retain the blade in position by the countertraction exerted by tissues. The blades are made in different shapes and lengths, thus allowing the surgeon to alter exposure in different parts of the wound as required.

In some operations, traction is required which may be beyond the average assistant's or retractor's ability. In vagotomy a particularly strong upward traction on the xiphisternum is required, and Goligher's sternal-lifting retractor was designed for just this purpose. It consists of two vertical bars fixed to the table on each side of the patient and connected by a transverse bar at their top end. A hook attached to a chain is placed under the xiphisternum and the chain, under tension, is hooked over the transverse bar, thus maintaining a continuous upward retraction. This retractor is unpopular with anaesthetists.

8.10 Cholecystectomy instruments

Cholecystectomy has been an established surgical procedure for benign and malignant conditions of the gall bladder for over 100 years. It is the most commonly performed major elective abdominal operation.

Good exposure is necessary for successful surgery and this is especially so in cholecystectomy. A good assistant and a good retractor, such as the Kelly, are essential.

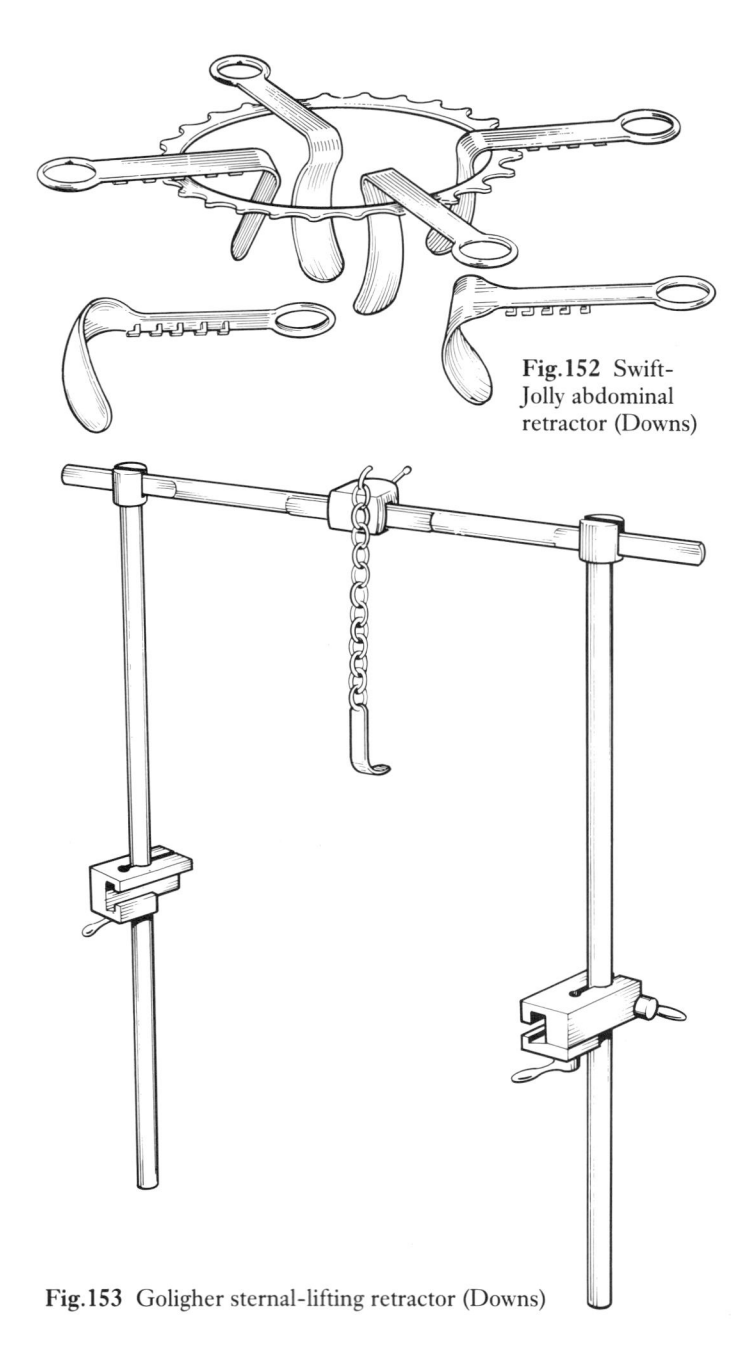

Fig.152 Swift-Jolly abdominal retractor (Downs)

Fig.153 Goligher sternal-lifting retractor (Downs)

The gall bladder may be so large as to obscure the operative field. If it is distended with bile, a cannula and trochar can be used with or without suction or, simply, a hypodermic needle and syringe.

In simple cholecystostomy for empyema, gall stones may be scooped out with a gall stone scoop into Mayo's gall stone spoon.

Gall-bladder forceps are designed to grip the gall bladder and allow its manipulation. Perhaps the most popular are Moynihan's. These are long, robust, curved forceps with a transverse serration for secure grip. They are, however, too coarse to be used for the dissection of the cystic duct.

Lahey forceps are much more versatile. Their jaws are slender and more acutely curved with fine, although blunt, tips. These forceps can be usefully employed for blunt dissection, for passing a ligature round the cystic artery and duct and for clamping the cystic duct. Any slender, long scissors are suitable, especially Metzenbaum's or Nelson's.

Exploration of the common bile duct requires forceps for blind location and removal of stones. Desjardins forceps have long slender jaws with a choice of curves. The jaws are fenestrated to reduce the distance between them when a stone is gripped in the confined space of the bile ducts. Alternatively, stones can be scooped out with a Cheatle gall stone scoop or the flexible Desjardins scoop.

Various probes have been designed

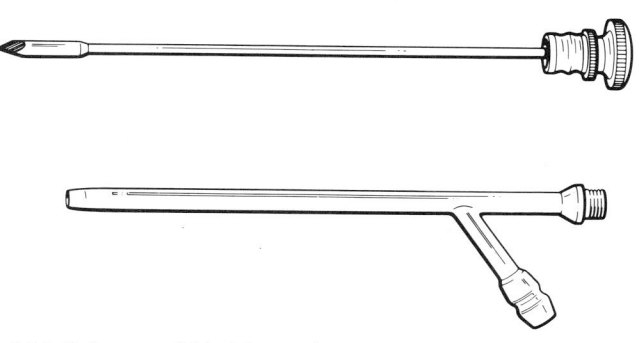

Fig.154 Ochsner gall bladder trochar

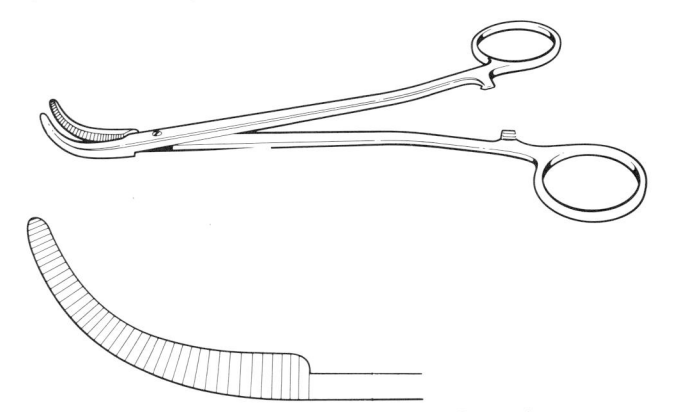

Fig.155 Moynihan cholecystectomy forceps (Downs)

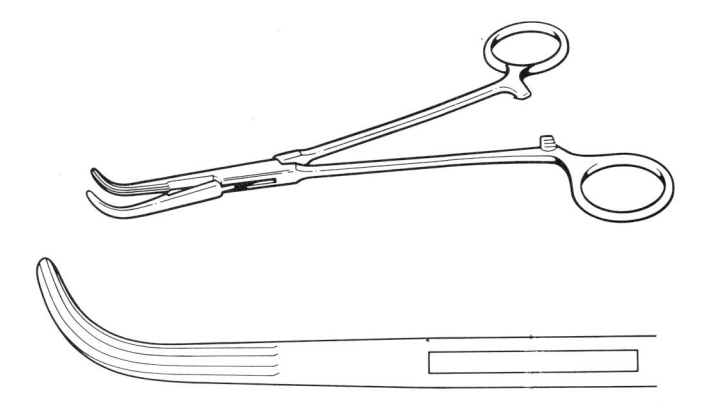

Fig.156 Lahey cholecystectomy forceps (Downs)

for testing the patency of the intersphincteric part of the common bile duct. Bakes dilators are olive-shaped and 3–11 mm in diameter, with a slender, malleable shaft and round handle. In spite of being blunt they are often responsible for a false passage being made into the duodenum when the sphincteric part of the common bile duct is obstructed or too narrow.

8.11 Thyroid instruments

Thyroidectomy has a long-established place in general surgery. Some instruments were developed specifically to facilitate this apparently simple surgical procedure. Access is, as ever, very important. The skin flaps of thyroidectomy incision must be retracted to provide unhindered access without obscuring the surgeon's view.

Joll's thyroidectomy skin retractor is more frequently used than Kocher's or Mayo's because the skin edges cannot slip off and retraction is more sensitively controlled by the screw-type retaining mechanism than by the ratchet-type. Lateral retraction of strap muscles can be achieved by a Langenbeck-type hand retractor, although Joll used his own device.

For ligature of vessels and pedicles a set of aneurysm needles should be available.

Kocher's dissector, or goitre enucleator, is now used only for the isolation of the superior thyroid pedicle. The instrument having been passed behind the pedicle, an

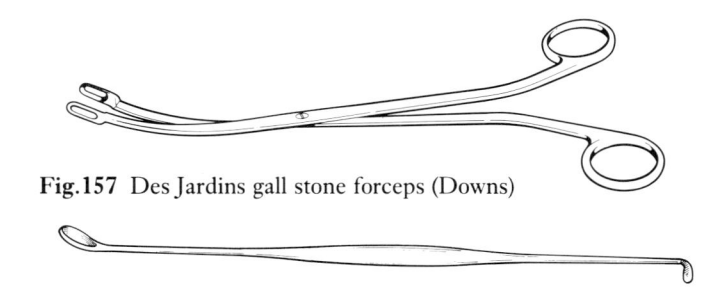

Fig.157 Des Jardins gall stone forceps (Downs)

Fig.158 Cheatle gall stone scoop (Downs)

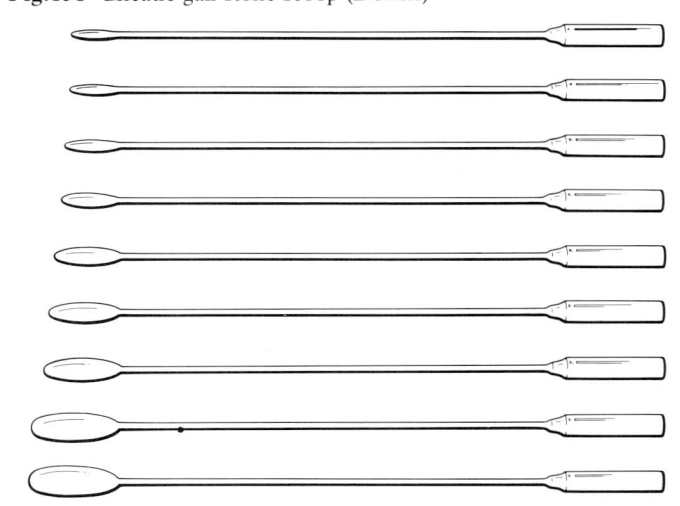

Fig.159 Bakes bile duct dilators (Downs)

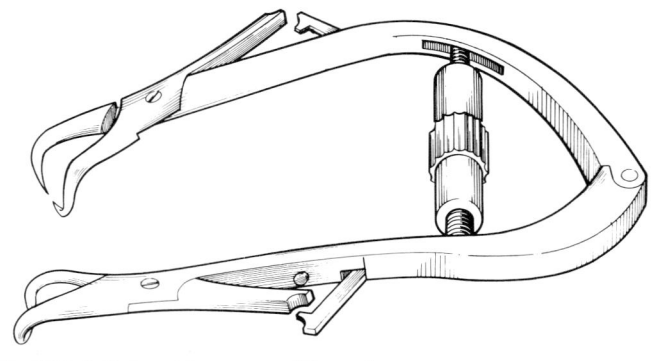

Fig.160 Joll thyroid retractor (Downs)

aneurysm needle can be passed between it and the pedicle. A large number of fine artery forceps will be required.

Finally, many still favour skin closure with Michel clips. These are V-shaped before application. The magazine holding the clips is held in the left hand and tenaculum forceps in the right hand. Clips are removed from the magazine one by one and compressed on to the skin edges using the tenaculum forceps. The clips can easily be removed by extraction forceps, which flatten the clip in the middle.

Rundle, F.F. (1951) *Joll's Diseases of the Thyroid Gland*, 2nd edn. Heinemann, London.

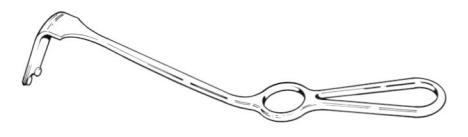

Fig.161 Joll retractor (Downs)

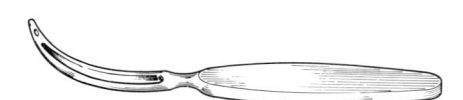

Fig.162 Kocher thyroid dissector (Downs)

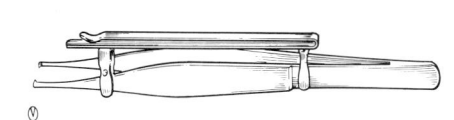

Fig.165 Michel skin-holding forceps (Downs)

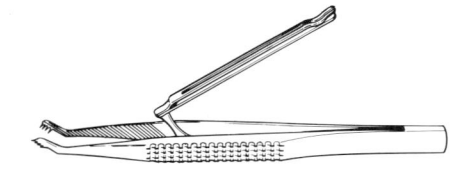

Fig.166 Childe skin-holding forceps (Downs)

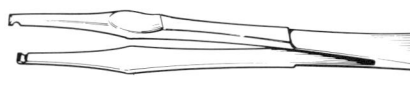

Fig.167 Michel clip-applying forceps (Downs)

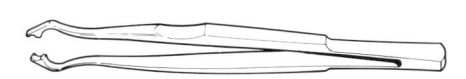

Fig.168 Kifa clip-applying forceps (Downs)

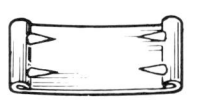

Fig.163 Michel clip (Downs)

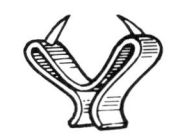

Fig.164 Kifa clip (Downs)

Chapter 9   Gastrointestinal Stapling Instruments

Anastomotic dehiscence in gastrointestinal and colonic surgery is accompanied by high morbidity and mortality. Consequently, for more than a century, surgeons have strived for a safe method of anastomosis.

The idea of mechanical stapling in intestinal anastomosis, in place of sutures, is not new. The principles of inverting intestinal suture were established by Lembert in 1826. In the same year, Denans of Marseilles developed a mechanical method of end-to-end anastomosis which represents the first serious attempt at mechanical anastomosis without sutures. The device used consisted of two silver rings over which the bowel ends were invaginated and the two rings were then approximated by a hollow spring within the ring's lumen. the result was a full-thickness, inverted, end-to-end anastomosis. However, the rings occasionally impacted inside the bowel, instead of being passed spontaneously.

Intraluminal stents became fashionable at that time and various materials, including trachea and cork, were used for this purpose. Halsted showed experimentally that Lembert's technique was acceptably safe, providing that submucosa was included in the suture.

In 1892 Benjamin Murphy described an anastomotic button which was originally designed for cholecystojejunostomy. The button was based on the same principle as Denans's rings and suffered from the same problem, namely intraluminal impaction.

Intraperitoneal colonic anastomosis continued to be the source of dehiscence in large number of cases and for that reason exteriorisation of colon became a popular practice. It was made popular by Bloch, Paul and von Mikulicz. The bridge of apposed ends of the colon was crushed with an enterotome.

Parker and Kerr popularised the aseptic closed method of anastomosis.

The first stapling instrument was developed by Hültl in 1908 but it was complex and very heavy. It placed four rows of staples, so that stomach and duodenum could be transected. De Petz described a stapling instrument in 1921 which was simpler and lighter. It was also designed for gastrectomy. The lumen of the stomach was closed by two rows of B-shaped staples. After World War II, Androsov in Russia developed stapling instruments for blood vessel anastomosis and these were later modified for intestinal anastomosis.

In 1960 the Russians developed a gun-like stapling machine (PKS-25) which, introduced intraluminally, produced an end-to-end inverted oesophago-jejunal anastomosis. Subsequent development of this instrument resulted in the KTs-28, which was used in colorectal anastomosis and later developed into the now famous SPTU gun.

In 1963 Hallenbeck, and two years later Brummelkamp, described a device for end-to-end colorectal anastomosis in anterior resection of the rectum. These instruments were however overshadowed by the subsequent introduction of the SPTU and EEA devices. In 1970 Boerema described a device for transection of the oesophagus for varices (Boerema button).

There is no doubt that the Russians were the first to develop stapling instruments which were practical to use in surgery. However, it was the United States Surgical Corporation which developed these instruments further, making them truly disposable, reliable and easy to use. Since the USSC instruments are the most popular in the Western World they will be described in the following text. Although introduced as late as 1967, the circular EEA stapling gun is the most popular of the Auto-Suture instruments. EEA is an abbreviation for end-to-end anastomosis. It consists of a central shaft enclosed in a barrel. Proximally, the wing nut controls approximation and separation of the anvil and cartridge. The trigger lever drives the circular knife which trims the inverted bowel ends and, at the same time drives two rows of staples through the full thickness of the bowel. The stapling head consists of a cartridge and anvil. The cartridge is advanced over the central shaft along a grooved track and is locked into position on the cartridge carrier at the end of the barrel. The anvil is screwed on to the tip of the central rod. The cartridges are available in three sizes: 25, 28 and 31 mm.

Prior to its insertion a purse string is applied to both free ends of the bowel.

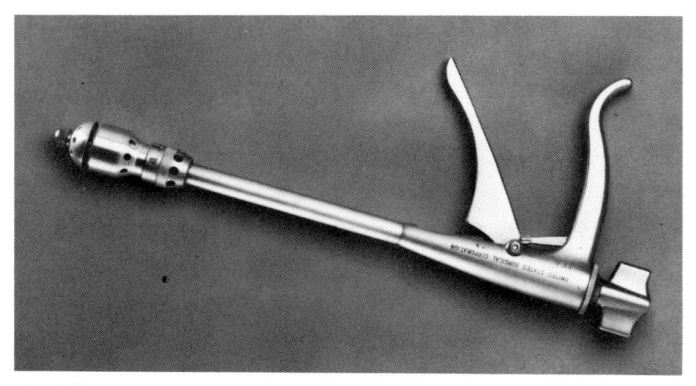

Fig.169 EEA stapling gun (Auto Suture)

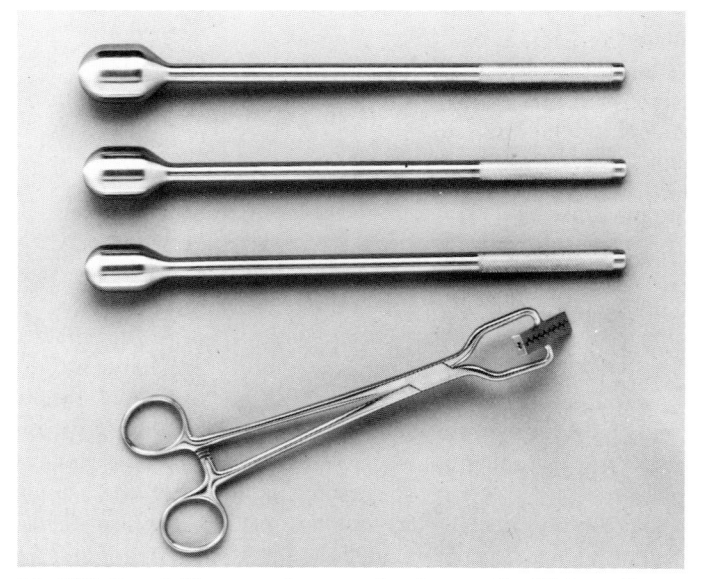

Fig.170 Bowel dilators and pursestring forceps for EEA stapling (Auto Suture)

The assembled instrument, with the anvil and cartridge approximated, is then inserted into the bowel lumen. When the anvil appears through the bowel end the wing nut is turned anticlockwise, resulting in the anvil separating from the cartridge. The purse string is tied firmly on to the shaft. The opposite bowel end is then manipulated over the anvil and the purse string tied so that the anvil is completely enclosed by the bowel. The wing nut is turned clockwise until both ends are approximated, as indicated by a gauge on the barrel. The gun is now ready for firing. The safety catch is released and the trigger level approximated to the handle. To remove the stapler the anvil is opened away from the cartridge, the gun is rotated and gently pulled out. The result is an end-to-end, inverted haemostatic anastomosis with two rows of staples. The disposable circular guns are exactly the same, except in the arrangement of the handle and firing lever. They are coded with a letter D (DEEA). The curved EEA stapler is specifically designed for oesophageal anastomosis (CDEEA). The gently curved barrel facilitates its per-oral or abdominal insertion. The TA (thoraco-abdominal) stapling instruments produce linear suture lines with a double, staggered row of staples. They are supplied in three sizes: 30, 55 and 90 mm in length. The instrument consists of a L-shaped frame, with the disposable anvil fixed onto the short limb of the L. The cartridge is slipped onto a jaw which slides along the shaft. The new generation of TA instruments utilise a lever, rather than a wing nut, for approximation of the cartridge to the anvil. A squeeze of the trigger lever drives the staples in. The older

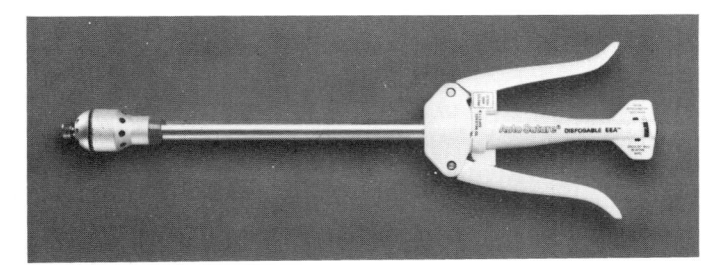

Fig.171 Disposable EEA stapling gun (Auto Suture)

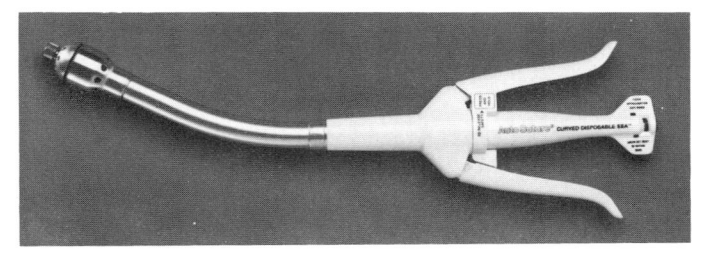

Fig.172 Curved disposable EEA gun (Auto Suture)

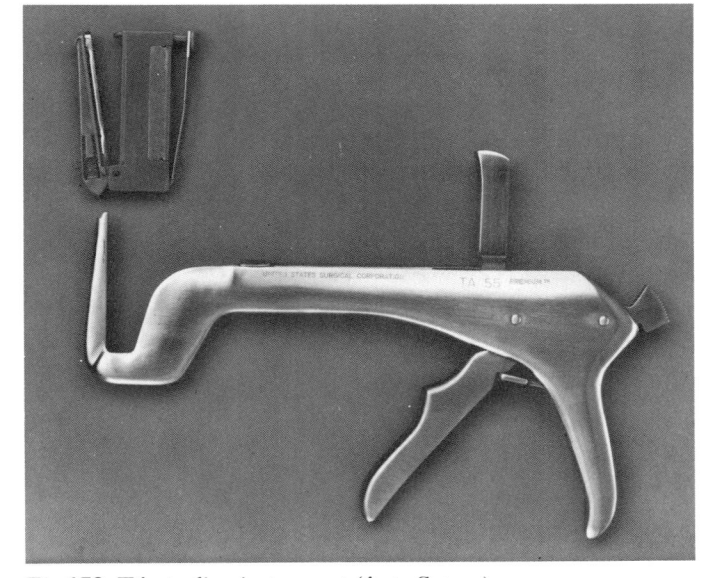

Fig.173 TA stapling instrument (Auto Suture)

generation TA instruments employed a pin between the anvil and the cartridge to prevent tissue from being squeezed outside the jaw and ensuring perfect alignment of cartridge and anvil for precise closure of staples. This instrument is used for closure of cut ends of stomach or bowel and for closing linear bowel incisions. It is no longer used for end-to-end bowel anastomosis. The GIA (gastrointestinal anastomosis) instrument is made in one size. It consists of two parts, each with a narrow protruding limb; one for the cartridge and the other for the anvil. The cartridge delivers two double rows of staples. A central blade between the two driving blades divides the tissue between these two double rows. Graduations on the limbs serve to measure the size of the anastomosis. The limbs are inserted into the bowel separately and joined by a locking device. The three-pronged assembly is driven home and the pusher assembly is withdrawn. Pressure on the spring release unlocks the two limbs and both can be removed. The instrument is used for lateral anastomoses, such as gastrojejunostomy and entero-enterostomy. The remaining defect in the bowel can be closed with the TA instrument.

Finally, the LDS (ligating–dividing–stapling) instrument deserves a mention. The instrument consists of a disposable cartridge and a driving handle with a trigger lever. The cartridge contains up to 15 pairs of staples and a knife. Its distal end is in the form of a hook.

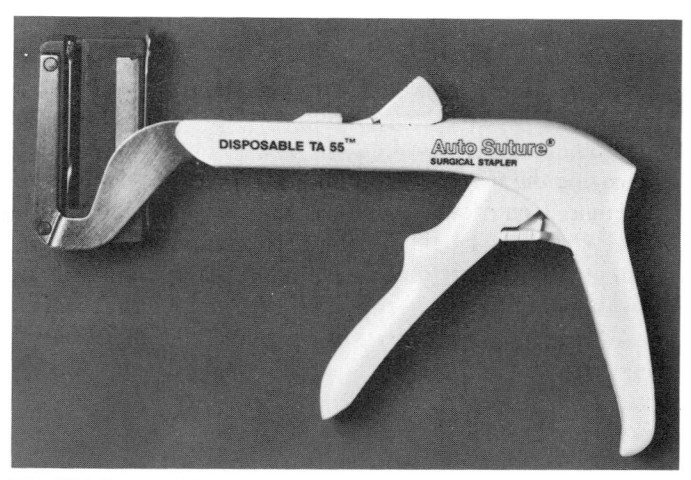

Fig. 174 Disposable TA stapling instrument (Auto Suture)

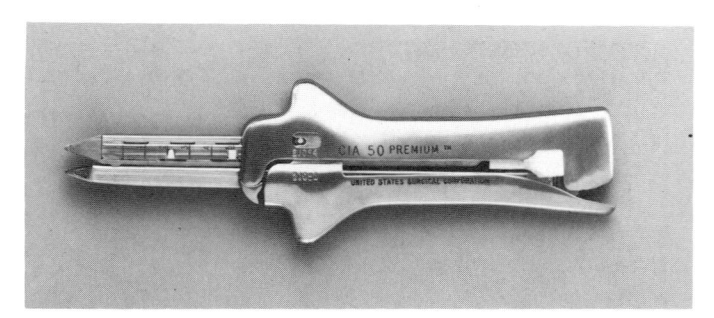

Fig. 175 GIA stapling instrument (Auto Suture)

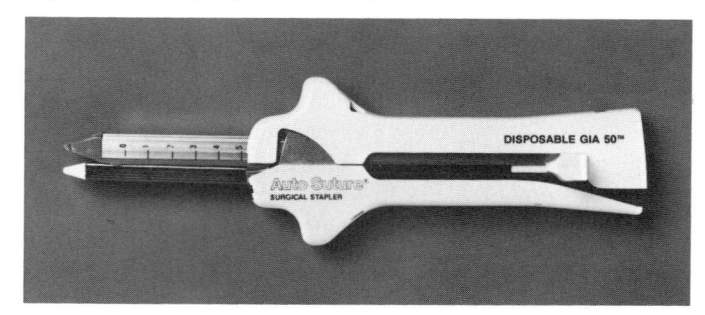

Fig. 176 Disposable GIA stapling instrument (Auto Suture)

It is used for ligation and division of pedicles and blood vessels. The pedicle is freed and the lip of the cartridge is hooked around it. The instrument is slightly withdrawn, thus engaging the tissue in the hook opening. Compression of the trigger lever closes the opening, staples compress the tissue on each side and the knife divides it.

All these instruments require experience in their use, otherwise considerable problems can be encountered. They are not suitable for experimenting, largely because of their prohibitive cost. However, when used selectively, they represent a revolutionary addition to the surgeon's armamentarium.

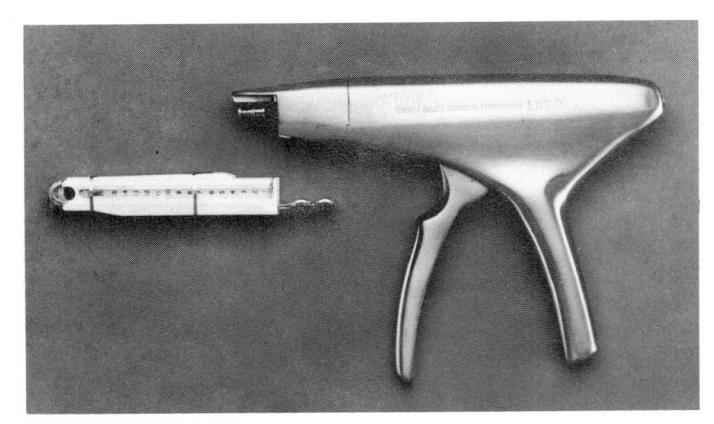

Fig.177 LDS stapling instrument (Auto Suture)

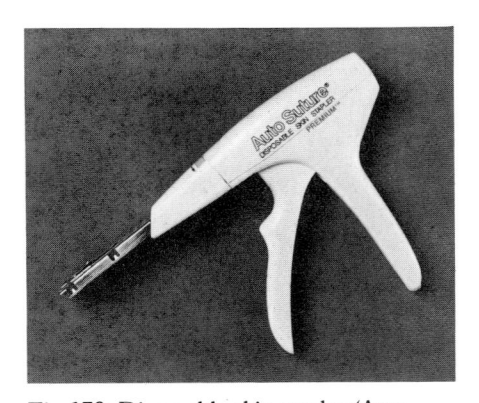

Fig.179 Disposable skin stapler (Auto Suture)

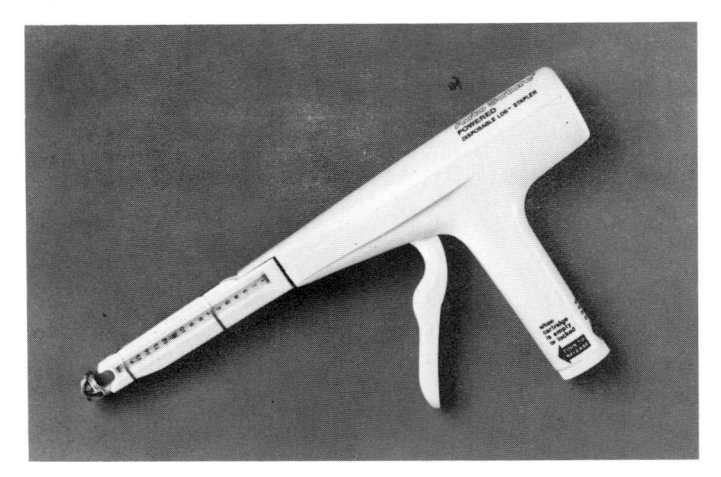

Fig.178 Disposable powered LDS stapling instrument (Auto Suture)

Fraser, I. (1982) An historical perspective on mechanical aids in intestinal anastomosis. *Surgery, Gynecology & Obstetrics*, **155**, 566-574.

De Petz, A. (1927) Aseptic technic of stomach resection. *Annals of Surgery*, **86**, 388-392.

Androsov, P.I. (1956) New method of surgical treatment of blood vessel lesions. *Archives of Surgery*, **73**, 902-910

Boerema, I., Klopper, P.F., Holscher, A.A. (1970) Transabdominal ligation-resection of the oesophagus in cases of bleeding oesophageal varices. *Surgery*, **67**, 409-413.

Hallenbeck, G.A., Judd, E.D. and David,

C. (1963) An instrument for colorectal anastomosis without sutures. *Diseases of Colon and Rectum*, **6**, 98-101.

Brummelkamp, R. (1965) The rectoresector: a new instrument for resection of the rectum and colorectal anastomosis without sutures. *Diseases of Colon and Rectum*, **8**, 49-51.

Steichen, F.M. and Ravitch, M.M. (1973) Mechanical sutures in surgery. *British Journal of Surgery*, **60**, 191-197.

Fazio, V.W. (1980) Colorectal anastomosis using the EEA stapler. Current surgical techniques 1980; 3, No 3, Schering Corporation.

Ravitch, M.M. and Steichen, F.M. (1972) Technics of staple suturing in the gastrointestinal tract. *Annals of Surgery*, **175**, 815-837.

Stapling Techniques: General Surgery, 2nd edn. (1980). United States Surgical Corporation.

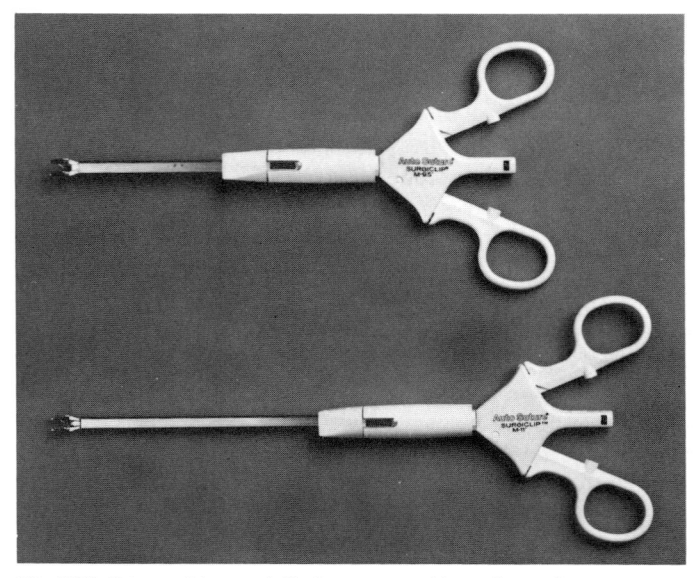

Fig.180 Disposable surgiclip instrument (Auto Suture)

Chapter 10 Plastic Surgery

10.1 Needle holders
10.2 Tissue forceps
10.3 Skin retractors
10.4 Dermatomes
10.5 Microsurgical instruments
10.6 Operating microscopes

10.1 Needle holders

Plastic surgery, whether reconstructive or cosmetic, deals largely with skin suturing, often using delicate needles and suture materials. One of the tasks of a plastic surgeon is to ensure that the scar is cosmetically unobstrusive. Most plastic needle holders are designed for skin suturing. For that reason they are short and delicate, and may have scissors incorporated.

The most well known plastic needle holder is Gillies. It resembles a pair of scissors with needle holder jaws instead of tips. The handles, one short for the thumb and one longer for the middle finger, have no ratchet to allow gentler handling of the needle and instrumental knot-tying.

In the original instrument, the jaws were oval in shape and fairly wide. One jaw had a longitudinal through-and-through slot and the opposite jaw had a groove on its inner aspect, directly opposite. This was to allow the placement of a suture needle in the long axis of the jaws, should it be required. The opposing surfaces of the jaws are cross-hatched to prevent the needle from slipping. The more recent Gillies needle holders have slimmer and more pointed jaws which make instrumental knot-tying easier. They are also slightly curved, with the convex surface facing the skin. Between the joint and the jaws are cutting blades, allowing the surgeon to cut his own suture.

Foster's needle holder is a miniature Gillies needle holder, suitable for finer needles and suture materials.

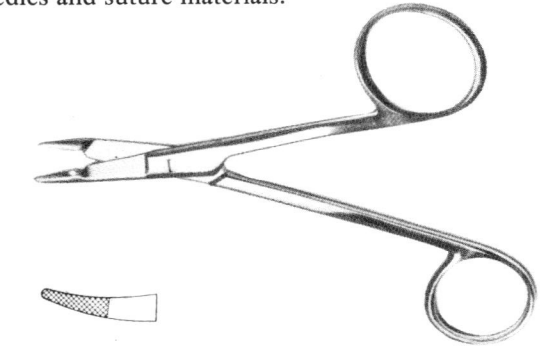

Fig.182 Foster needle holder (Downs)

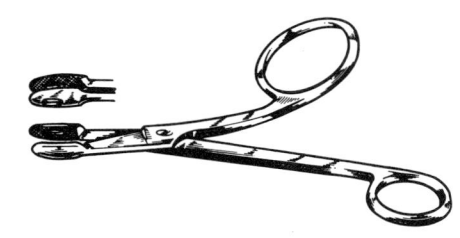

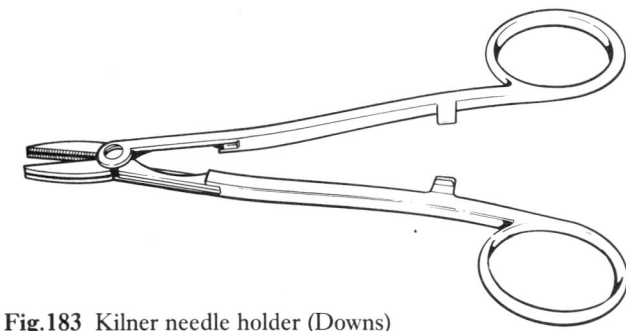

Fig.181 Gillies suture scissors and needle holder (Downs)

Fig.183 Kilner needle holder (Downs)

Another needle holder, designed by Kilner, has laminated jaws which are more springy and are thus suitable for handling delicate needles. Another Kilner-type needle holder has handles with a ratchet curved away from the operating surface. The jaws form a smooth line with the box joint, preventing suture from being caught during knot-tying.

10.2 Tissue forceps

Careful handling of skin edges and tissues is one of the arts of plastic surgery. The formation of a fine scar is determined not only by careful placement of sutures without tension but also by good blood supply to the skin edges. For that reason, dissecting forceps have fine tips and minimal force is required to close them. Although toothed forceps are designed primarily for skin suturing, it should be remembered that they puncture the skin and produce tissue oedema.

Non-toothed forceps are used primarily for dissection of fine structures such as nerves or arteries. Adson's dissecting forceps, toothed and non-toothed, are the most popular in plastic surgery. They are fine and short, and provide a large contact for thumb and index finger, being consequently more sensitive.

McIndoe's forceps are longer and narrower although equally fine. They are characterised by a pin half-way between the jaws which prevents excessive pressure from being applied, as well as preventing lateral misalignment of the jaws.

10.3 Skin retractors

There is no place for indelicate instruments when it comes to manipulating skin, as when undermining, excising a dog-ear or creating a Z-plasty. Skin edges are sensitive to any degree of ischaemia, especially if part of a flap, which may result in devitalisation, delayed healing and an ugly scar. For that reason plastic surgeons use very fine, usually

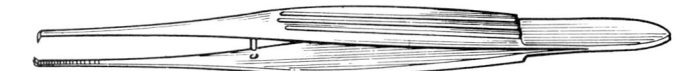

Fig.186 McIndoe dissecting forceps (Downs)

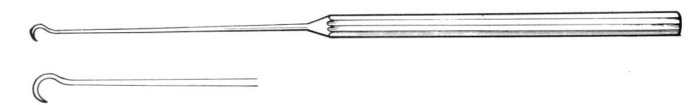

Fig.187 Gillies skin hook (Downs)

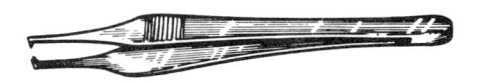

Fig.184 Adson toothed forceps (Downs)

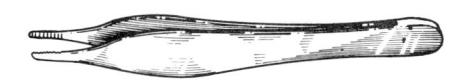

Fig.185 Adson non-toothed forceps (Downs)

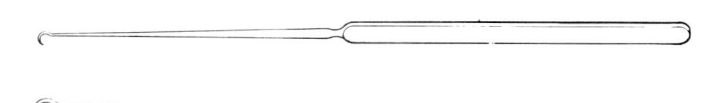

Fig.188 McIndoe skin hook (Downs)

PLASTIC SURGERY 111

hand-held, retractors. They are exemplified by the Gillies fine skin hook and similar devices, such as the Kilner retractor and McIndoe hook.

Apart from the slim handle, the shaft of the hook is slender and tapering. The hook itself is fine and needle-sharp. It is never hooked through the skin but always through subcutaneous tissue, whether lifting, retracting or stretching the skin edges.

The Gordon hook has the advantage that it is self-retaining; the hook is attached to a weight by a chain. Fine skin hooks are also invaluable for accurate placing and holding of free grafts.

Less delicate retractors, also suitable for skin work, usually have two or three hooks, as exemplified by the Kilner skin retractor or the McIndoe double skin hook.

There are several delicate, self-retaining retractors suitable for small skin incisions. The Kilner small skin retractor is made of a stainless steel spring with a double hook on each jaw.

The Alms self-retaining skin retractor has fine spikes on the end of two arms which are approximated or retracted by means of screw-operated hinged arms.

10.4 Dermatomes

Grafting of free skin is an established technique for providing cover where skin has been lost. While whole skin grafts can be removed with the use of a scalpel, the removal of a split skin graft requires the use of a dermatome.

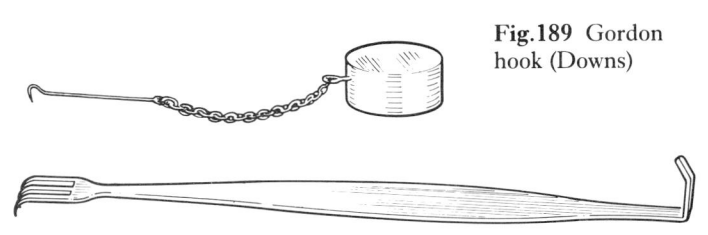

Fig.189 Gordon hook (Downs)

Fig.190 Kilner skin retractor (Downs)

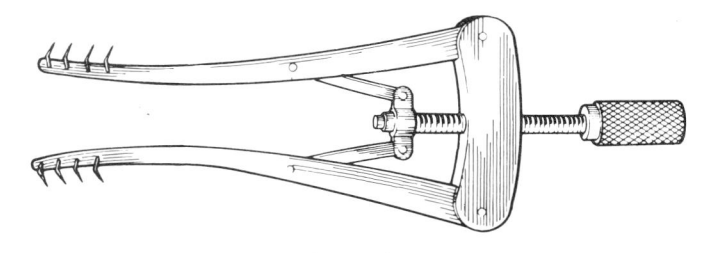

Fig.191 Alms skin retractor (Downs)

The Blair knife was the first knife specifically designed for removal of split skin graft and is now rarely used. It is a long, straight-edged knife with a handle. Its disadvantage is the extreme difficulty of cutting a graft of correct and even thickness.

The Blair knife has been replaced by the Humby pattern knife. This also has a long, straight-edged blade, usually detachable, and a handle. The

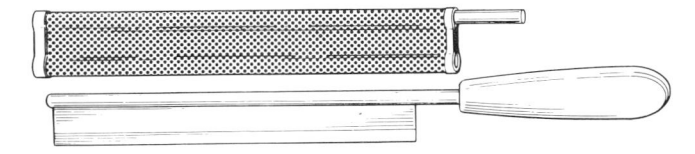

Fig.192 Blair skin-grafting knife (Downs)

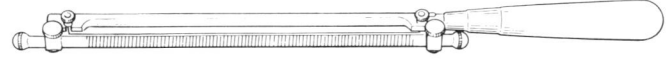

Fig.193 Humby skin-grafting knife (Downs)

modification is the addition of an adjustable roller which allows control of graft thickness, by adjustment of the distance between roller and blade. Adjustment settings on the knife are unreliable and the best way to assess the actual clearance between the knife edge and the roller is by holding the knife up to the light.

To facilitate graft cutting, the skin is made taught with a wooden board which also makes the surface flat. The edge of the board is lubricated with liquid paraffin so that it can advance steadily with the knife. The knife is placed flat on the skin, and to-and-fro motion initiates cutting. The drum dermatome, such as the Padgett, is used infrequently. It consists of a half-drum, a central handle and a knife. The knife lies parallel to the convex surface of the drum and can be moved along its surface by its attachment to the central handle by two lateral bars.

By adjusting the distance between the blade and the drum surface the thickness of the graft is selected. The drum and donor areas are painted with an adhesive compound and the drum is pressed against the skin so that both surfaces adhere and the skin can be lifted. The knife is then pressed against the skin edge and cutting is initiated by to-and-fro movement of the knife side handle, parallel to the axis of the drum. The graft is left adhering to the drum.

The electric dermatome is not unlike a large electric hair cutter. The cutting blade oscillates rapidly, being driven by electricity or compressed air.

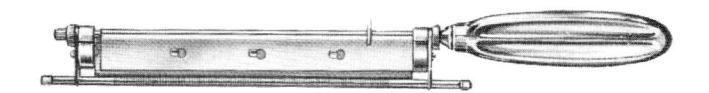

Fig.194 Braithwaite modification of Humby knife (Downs)

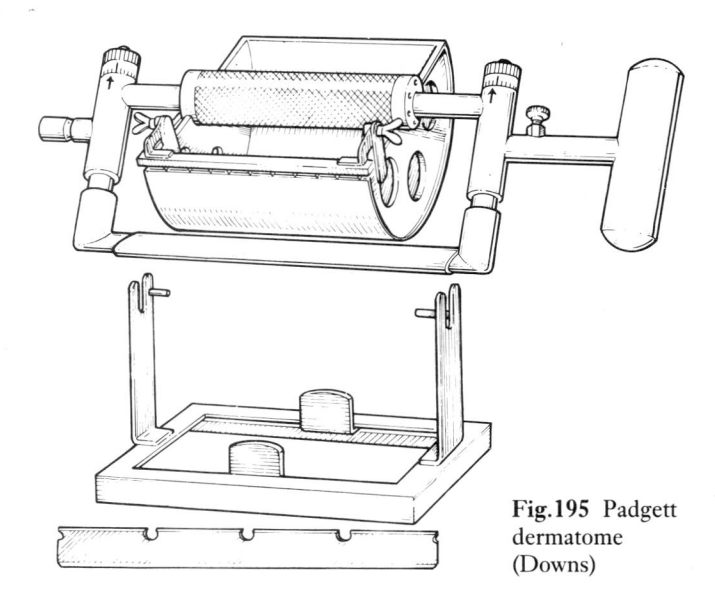

Fig.195 Padgett dermatome (Downs)

It too has an adjustable roller which controls the graft thickness. It is particularly suitable when large areas of skin are to be cut, as in extensive deep burns. One of its advantages is that the thickness of graft is accurate and thin grafts are easily obtained from most parts of the body.

Because of the straight margin and uniform thickness, a whole limb can be flayed without any wastage and re-used for further grafting when the donor area is healed.

Humby, G. (1934) Apparatus for skin graft cutting. *British Medical Journal* 1934, **1**, 1078.

10.5 Microsurgical instruments

Microsurgery deals with structures which cannot be adequately seen without some kind of magnification. It particularly applies to surgery of small blood vessels, nerves, eye and ear.

Microsurgical instruments are small and very precise. Nyler was first to use a modified microscope for middle ear surgery in 1921 and since the late 1950s microsurgery has been applied to microvascular and microneural anastomoses.

The potential of microsurgery is vast and is continually expanding. The essential instruments are an operating microscope (section 10.6), a set of precise tools and fine sutures. The microsurgical instruments must be fine but not necessarily small. Forceps are non-toothed with fine points and are graded by numbers according to their fineness. No. 7 forceps can be used as needle holders.

Scissors are sharp-pointed, flat or curved, straight or angled. They all are spring-handled for precise action. Needle holders too are spring-handled, with fine jaws to avoid damage to fine needles. Many clamps are available for microvascular anastomoses and the most commonly used are those of the Acland type. These are flat clamps and some of them may have fine serrations on the inner surface to prevent the clamp from slipping.

Needles are 30–140 µm thick with taper, spatula or triangular points. The

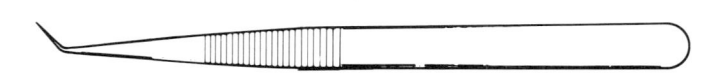

Fig.196 Microvascular forceps (Downs)

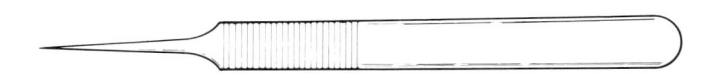

Fig.197 Microvascular forceps (Downs)

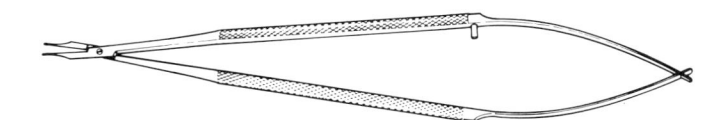

Fig.198 Microvascular needle holders (Downs)

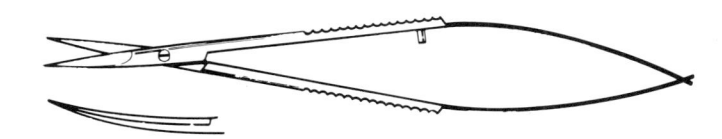

Fig.199 Microvascular dissecting scissors (Downs)

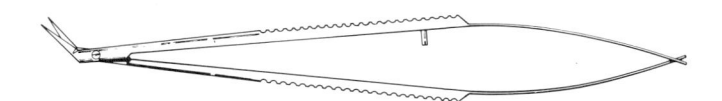

Fig.200 Microvascular dissecting scissors (Downs)

Fig.201 Acland single clamp (Downs)

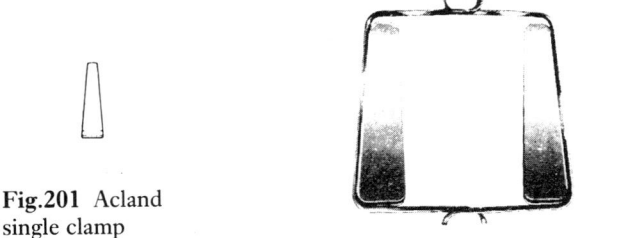

Fig.202 Acland double clamp (Downs)

suture material is usually nylon or silk of sizes 8−12 (0.4−0.1 metric).

Browning, F.S.C. (1979) Microsurgery. *Surgical Review 1* (ed. Lumley, J. and Craven, J.), p. 376. Pitman Medical, London.

10.6 Operating microscopes

Without the modern operating microscope, current ophthalmic, ENT and microvascular techniques would be unthinkable. Although the slit-lámp microscope was first used in the 1920s for eye and ear surgery, it was not until 1953 that Zeiss produced the first operating microscope, the now famous Opmi 1.

A system which magnifies between 2× and 8× is known as visual aid. Providing that the field of vision is adequately illuminated the minimum requirements for visual aid are an enlarged image, which must be unreversed and two-dimensional, and a working distance of at least 150 mm.

In microsurgery the use of prism loupes is limited by a maximum useful magnification. Since the prism loupes follow the movement of the head, this leads to blurring of the image which becomes worse with increasing speed of movement. A further disadvantage is the fixed focal length, which requires the surgeon to keep his head at a fixed distance from the operation site.

Moreover, the illumination may be poor, especially at higher magnification. This problem can be partially overcome by the use of a

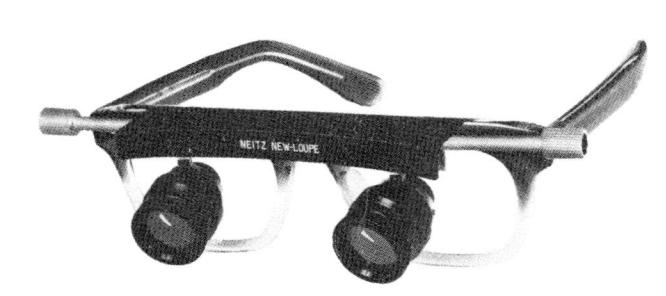

Fig.203 Downs Neitz binocular loupe BL-1

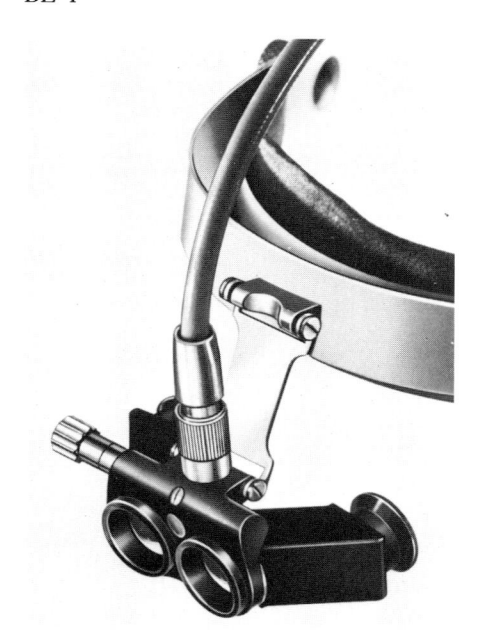

Fig.204 Prism loupe with fibrelight source (Storz)

headlamp but this can make the equipment very expensive.

The operating microscope provides a visual aid without the disadvantage of a prism loupe with many additional requirements. Magnifications up to 60× may have to be used, and microsurgical techniques require more than one magnification. Equally, the optimum working distance varies from operation to operation and from surgeon to surgeon. Image quality becomes very important with increasing magnification, and a wide range of depth of focus is necessary. Illumination also becomes important at higher magnifications, and a co-axial illumination system, which illuminates the operating field through the microscope, is a prerequisite for microsurgery.

There should be provision for an assistant's eyepiece, which offers the same view of the operating field. The microscope should have a safe and stable mounting, and be easily adjustable, preferably by remote control.

Holmgren, G. (1923) Some experiences in the surgery of otosclerosis. *Acta Oto-laryngologica*, **5**, 460.

Yasangil, M.G. (1969) *Microsurgery Applied to Neurosurgery*. Academic Press, New York.

Davies, C.H. (1981) Operating microscopes and magnification system. *British Journal of Hospital Medicine*, March 1981, 291-296.

Lang, W.H. and Michael, F. (1982) *Zeiss Microscopes of Microsurgery*. Springer-Verlag, Berlin.

Chapter 11   Urology

11.1 Urethral sounds and bougies
11.2 Urethrotome
11.3 Resectoscope
11.4 Lithotrite
11.5 Catheter introducers
11.6 Pyelolithotomy instruments
11.7 Prostatectomy instruments
11.8 Bladder evacuator
11.9 Ureteric basket stone extractors
11.10 Percutaneous pyelolithotomy

11.1 Urethral sounds and bougies

There is a lot of confusion surrounding the terminology of urethral dilating instruments. A sound is, strictly speaking, a solid rod of uniform bore and curved end which is used for the detection of bladder stones. A dilating sound looks like a stone sound but has a tapering shaft. A bougie is a solid, flexible rod used for urethral dilatation. A staff may resemble a bougie or a sound and has a groove on its surface. It is used to direct the knife in strictures.

Bladder stone sounds became obsolete with the advent of the diagnostic cystoscope. They resembled stricture sounds and had a long, cylindrical shaft, a large handle and a long terminal curve. The sound passed into the bladder and the presence of stones was detected by feeling a metallic contact transmitted to the surgeon's fingers via the long slender shaft.

The most commonly used dilating sounds are Lister's and Clutton's. These all taper gradually. Lister's dilating sounds have a longer curve than Clutton's and have a bulbous point. They are made in 12 sizes, 0–2 to 9–12 English gauge (a series of sizes gradually increasing by a diameter of 0.5 mm; 2 = 2 mm). The numbers refer to the diameter at the tip and shoulder respectively.

Clutton's dilating sounds were designed in 1888 and are made in French gauge sizes 14–18 to 28–32. They have a curved handle and blunt tip. The sound is passed into the urethra under its own weight, the convex surface of the curved end pointing towards the patient. When the bulbar urethra has been reached the instrument is rotated by 180°, so that the curve of the instrument can follow the natural curve of the urethra. By gently pressing down the handle, the instrument will enter the bladder.

Filiform bougies are thin and flexible gum elastic rods. They are used for particularly narrow strictures. Several may have to be passed parallel to each other before the stricture is

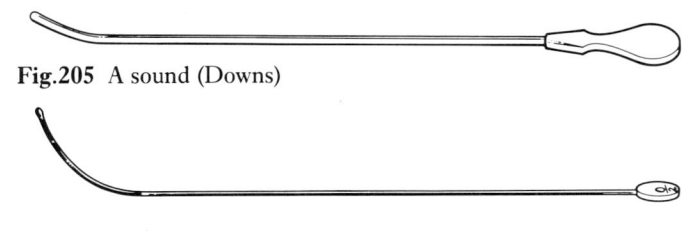

Fig.205 A sound (Downs)

Fig.206 Lister sound (Downs)

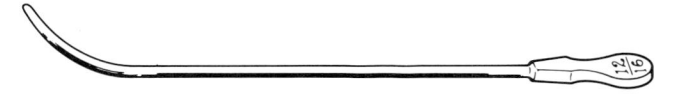

Fig.207 Clutton sound (Downs)

negotiated. The end of the filiform can be screwed into a metal dilating sound or a follower, and the stricture thus dilated.

The Wheelhouse staff was designed in 1870 for impassable strictures. It is a straight, grooved staff with a crochet-like hook at the tip which points in the opposite direction to the groove. The staff is passed with its grooved surface facing the ventral surface of the penis. When the stricture is reached the operator cuts down through the perineal skin into the groove and rotates the staff so that the hook appears through the wound and retracts its edge. The stricture then may be divided under direct vision using the Wheelhouse director.

11.2 Urethrotome

Internal urethrotomy for strictures has been practised for many centuries. Originally, most urethrotomes were effectively urethral catheters with sharp bistouries at the distal end. The real breakthrough in internal urethrotomy came with the introduction of the Otis urethrotome.

This instrument consists of two parallel blades hinged at the proximal end and connected by several hinged cross bars. A knob on the instrument's handle operates a screw which pushes or pulls the thinner, mobile blade. By pushing the blade towards the distal end the gap between the blades increases, being largest at the tip and smallest at the handle. The main blade has a groove on its upper aspect. This accepts the urethrotome knife, which

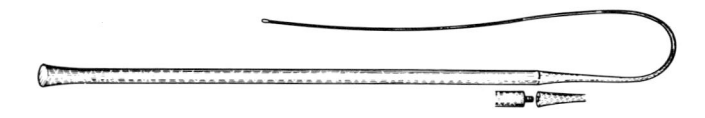

Fig.208 Canny Ryall bougie (Downs)

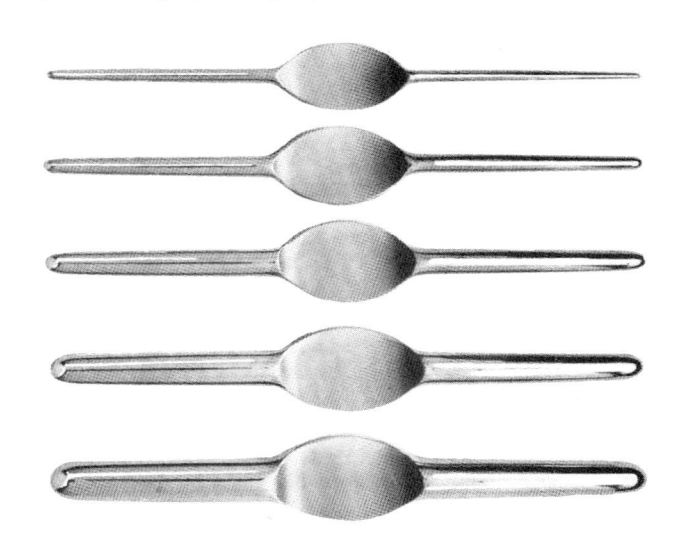

Fig.209 Turner Warwick bladder neck spreader (Downs)

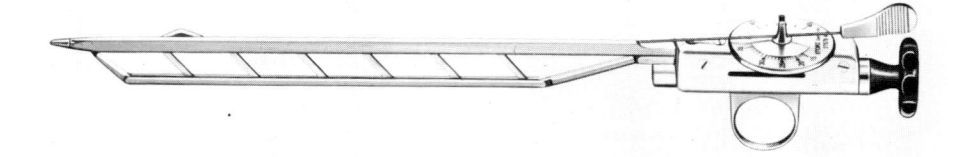

Fig.210 Otis urethrotome (modified) (Storz)

moves along the long axis of the instrument only. When the knife is at the tip its blade is completely hidden. It only protrudes by several millimetres when pulled proximally. A dial on top of the handle, calibrated in French gauge, indicates the maximum distance between the two blades.

The reason that the distal width is larger than the proximal is because Otis discovered that the bulbar urethra is larger than the rest of the urethra.

The urethrotome is passed through the stricture and opened until a distinct grip is felt. The knife is pulled against the strictures and the whole instrument is then withdrawn, knife and all. The result is a linear cut along the urethra, approximately 3 mm in depth. In cases of a difficult stricture, filiform bougies can be used for dilatation and the tip of the Otis urethrotome can be screwed to the last filiform as the follower and passed through the stricture.

Internal urethrotomy has been revolutionised by the optical urethrotomy, described by Sachse in 1974. The instrument is effectively a resectoscope with a 0° telescope and a cold knife instead of the cutting loop. There are obvious advantages in urethrotomy under direct vision. Even the most difficult strictures can be divided without the need for prior dilatation, which only traumatises the urethra. The procedure is quicker and safer because there is no need for blind instrumentation with false passages. However, there is no evidence that direct internal urethrotomy cures more urethral strictures than blind urethrotomy.

Blandy, J. (1978) *Transurethral Resection*, 2nd edn. Pitman Medical, London.
Blandy, J. (1978) *Operative Urology*. Blackwell Scientific Publications, Oxford.
Blandy, J. (1976) Urethral stricture and carcinoma. In: *Urology II* (ed. Blandy, J.). Blackwell Scientific Publications, Oxford.
Kirchheim, D., Tremann, J.A. and Ansell, J.S. (1978) Transurethral urethrotomy under vision. *Journal of Urology*, **119**, 496-499.
Engel, R.M.E., Wise, H.A. and Whitaker,

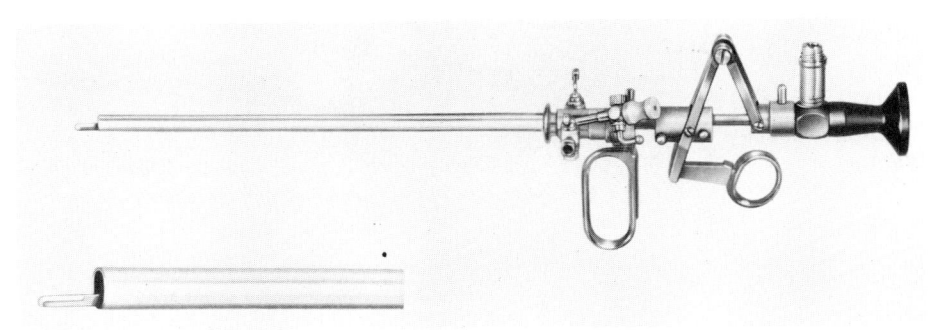

Fig.211 Storz optical urethrotome

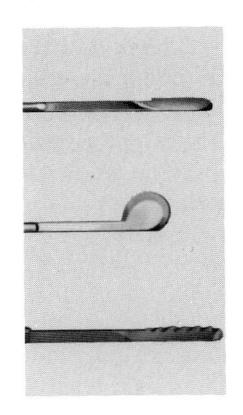

Fig.212 Optical urethrotome knives (Storz)

R.H. (1972) Otis internal urethrotomy with long-term urethral intubation. A comparison of latex and silastic catheters. *South African Medical Journal*, **65**, 55.

Attwater, H.L. (1973) The history of urethral stricture. *British Journal of Urology*, **15**, 39.

Sachse, H. (1974) Zur Behandlung der Harnröhrehstriktur die transurethrale Schlitzung unter Sicht mit Scharfem Schnitt. *Fortschritte der Medizin*, **42**, 12.

11.3 Resectoscope

The introduction of a transurethral resectoscope has altered the surgical approach to prostatectomy and management of superficial bladder tumours. Beer was the first to try a high-frequency diathermy current via a cystoscope for bladder papillomas. The introduction of valve diathermy and cutting current, together with improvements to the optical viewing system, led to the introduction of what is known as the Stern−McCarthy resectoscope. The modern instrument is more sophisticated, but remains essentially the same.

The beak of the resectoscope is made of insulating acrylic or melamine, or steel coated with Teflon, to prevent current being transmitted from the cutting loop into the resectoscope sheath.

Iglesias's two-way irrigating resectoscope has made transurethral resection of tumours and prostate easier because the constant volume of fluid in the bladder keeps the object of resection steady; constant dilution of

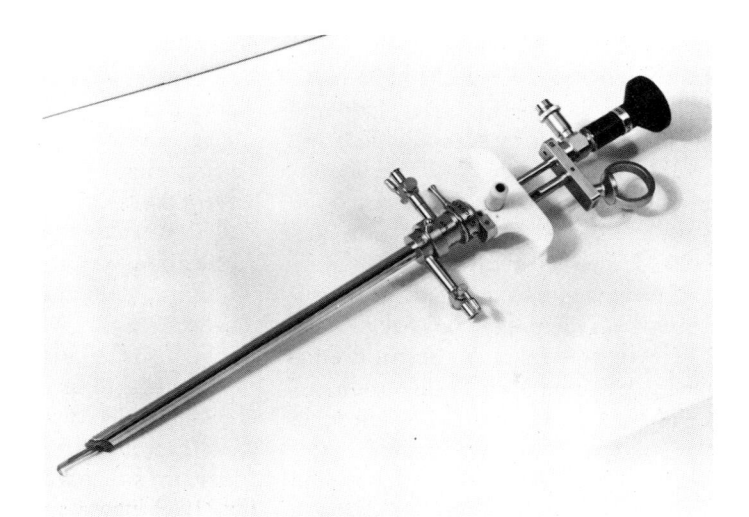

Fig.213 Olympus constant flow resectoscope (Key Med)

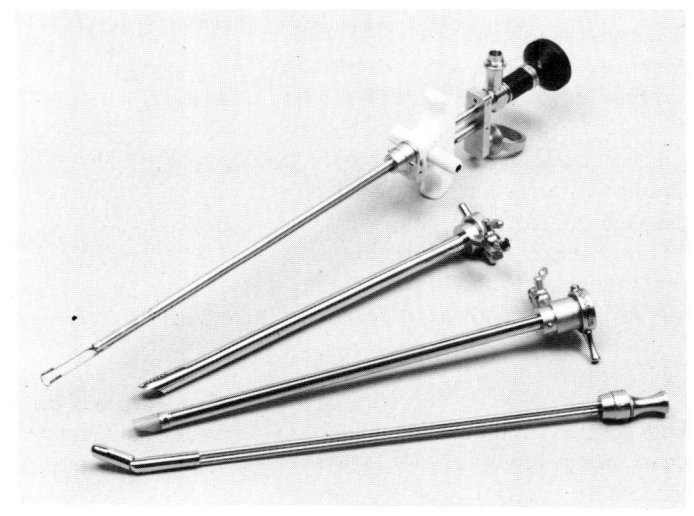

Fig.214 Components of Olympus constant flow resectoscope (Key Med)

blood improves definition and there is no need for frequent bladder emptying. The resectoscope sheath is double-skinned. The irrigating fluid is run in through the main lumen of the resectoscope sheath and outgoing fluid is aspirated at the same rate by a suction pump, through the channel between the outer and inner sheath.

The wire electrodes are insulated, except at the two ends. They are usually in the shape of a loop for cutting or as a ball for coagulation.

Blandy, J. (1978) *Transurethral Resection*, 2nd edn. Pitman Medical, London.
Stern, M. (1926) Resections of obstructions at the vesical orifice. *Journal of the Medical Association*, **87**, 1726.
McCarthy, J.F. (1931) A new apparatus for endoscopic plastic surgery of the prostate, diathermy and excision of vesical growths. *Journal of Urology*, **26**, 695.
Iglesias, J.J. (1975) New Iglesias resectoscope with simultaneous suction and continuous irrigation. *Endoscopy*, **7**, 36-40.

11.4 Lithotrite

The lithotrite is a tool for crushing urinary stones in the bladder. The first blind lithotrite, virtually as we know it, was made by Weiss of London in 1831, although the idea was originated by Civiale in Paris a few years earlier. Its introduction made lithotripsy, whether perineal or suprapubic, almost obsolete, except in the treatment of very large stones.

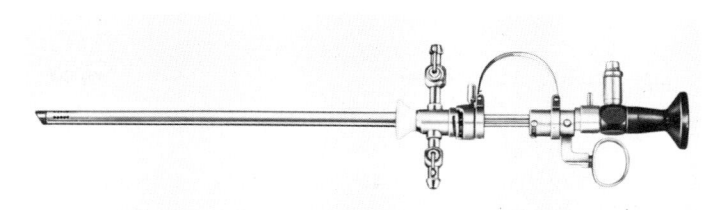

Fig.215 Iglesias two-way irrigating resectoscope (Storz)

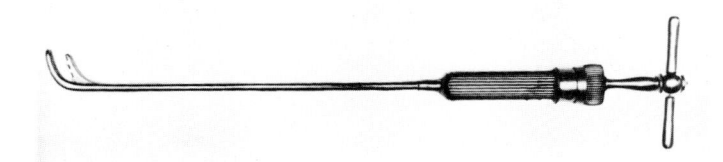

Fig.216 A lithotrite

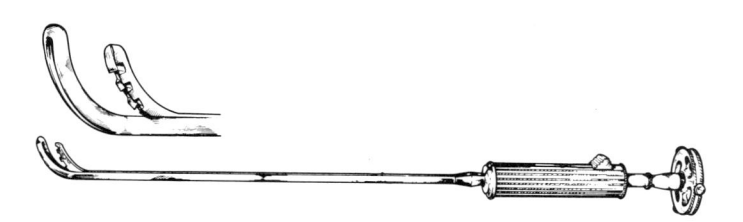

Fig.217 Thompson lithotrite (Downs)

Two types of blind lithotrite are in general use: the Freyer and Thompson patterns. They differ only in the mechanism and arrangement of the handle. The principle is simple; two fenestrated jaws are operated by a screw in a fixed handle. With the jaws closed the urethral part of the instrument resembles a sound. The female jaw is fixed to the handle while the male jaw can slide to and fro.

The lithotrite is passed with the jaws closed into a distended bladder. The

122 OPERATIVE INSTRUMENTS

jaws, pointing upwards, are then opened. The female jaw is pushed down onto the base of the bladder in order to allow the stone to roll between the jaws. The male blade grasps the stone and the jaws are lifted up to make sure that bladder wall has not been accidentally caught between them. The screw is then locked and by turning the wheel on the handle the stone is crushed. The procedure is then repeated for each of the fragments.

The optical lithotrite is essentially the same except that it has a telescope and fibrelight source which allow direct visualisation of both jaws in open and closed position. The jaws can be moved by a spring-loaded handle and crushing is achieved either by squeezing the handle or by turning a screw spindle. The telescopes used have a field of vision between 70° and 120°. An irrigating channel is provided. In contradistinction to the blind lithotrite, after insertion the jaws point towards the base of the bladder. The stone is gripped under direct vision and then crushed. The optical lithotrite is most suitable for smaller stones. Lithotripsy is contraindicated with existing urethral strictures, bladder diverticulae and stones which are fixed to the bladder wall. Injury to the urethra and bladder is the main hazard of this procedure.

Blandy, J. (1976) Stones and foreign bodies in the bladder. In: *Urology II* (ed. Blandy, J.), pp. 753-773. Blackwell Scientific Publications, Oxford.

Ellis, H. (1969) *A History of Bladder Stone.*

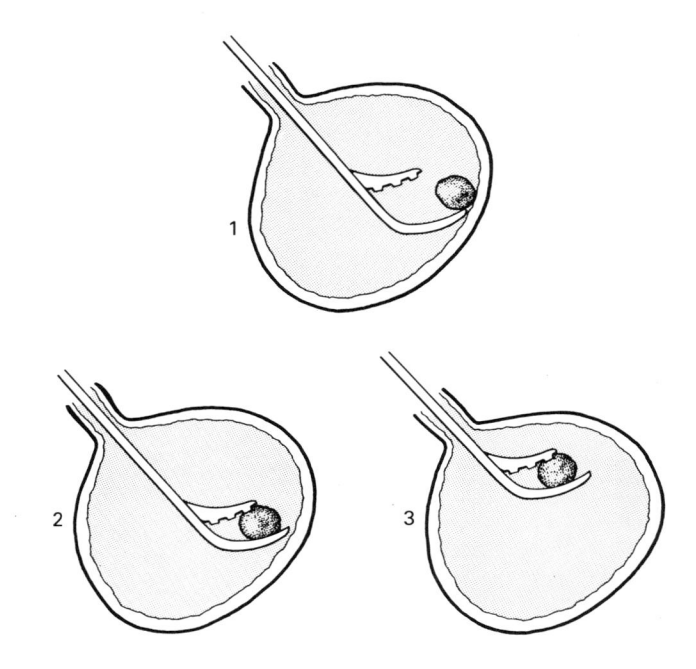

Fig.218 Blind lithotripsy

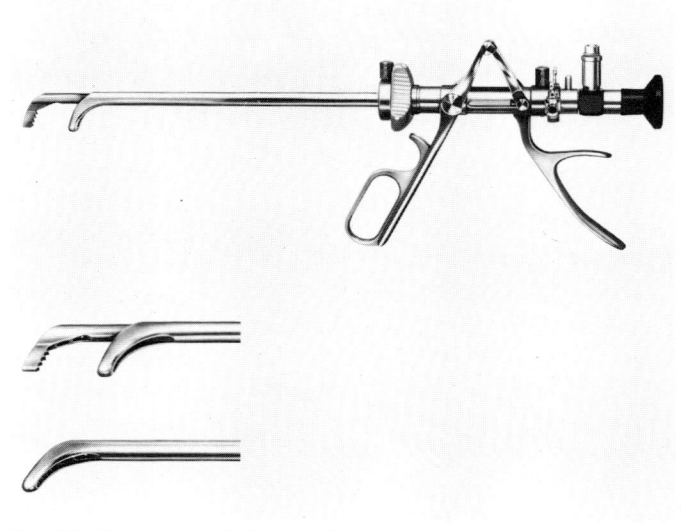

Fig.219 Storz optical lithotrite (Storz)

Blackwell Scientific Publications, Oxford.
Blandy, J. (1978) *Operative Urology.* Blackwell Scientific Publications, Oxford.

11.5 Catheter introducers

Soft urethral catheters may be difficult to insert into the male bladder for a variety of reasons. Other than urethral stricture the commonest cause of failure to pass the catheter is a relative obstruction of the prostatic urethra, especially when the middle lobe of the prostate is enlarged. This problem can be overcome by selecting a stiffer catheter or a coudé catheter. Following transurethral resection of prostate the catheter tip may curl up in the prostatic cavity and the balloon be inflated therein. However, soft catheters may be used in this situation by stiffening them with an introducer.

Wire stretchers can be inserted into the lumen of a Foley catheter and, after insertion into the bladder, removed. They are usually curved at the tip to allow negotiation of the prostatic urethra and the bladder neck.

Alternatively, a Maryfield introducer, described by Campbell and Douglas, can be used. The introducer is a curved metal tube whose convex wall has been removed. The tip is curved and pointed for insertion into the catheter tip. The catheter is stretched over the grooved convexity of the introducer and fixed under tension by a groove in the handle. After insertion the balloon is partially inflated and the introducer withdrawn.

The use of catheter introducers is fraught with danger of bladder perforation and urethral damage. This is especially so with the Maryfield introducer, which can slice the urethral wall during removal. Thus catheter introducers should be used only when conventional measures have failed and only by those who are skilled in their use and aware of the dangers involved.

Campbell, W. and Douglas, G. (1965) A new type of Foley catheter introducer. *Lancet*, 1965, **1**, 253

11.6 Pyelolithotomy instruments

Pyelolithotomy is a surgical procedure for removing pelvic or calyceal stones through an incision in the renal pelvis. It is unsuitable for very large stones, especially calyceal, when nephrolithotomy is more appropriate.

Gil-Vernet described a relatively bloodless approach to the posterior aspect of the renal pelvis and calyces through the intrasinusal plane. The entrance to the renal sinus is hidden by fat. By establishing a plane between the pelvis and adventitia with the fat, it is possible to enter the renal sinus

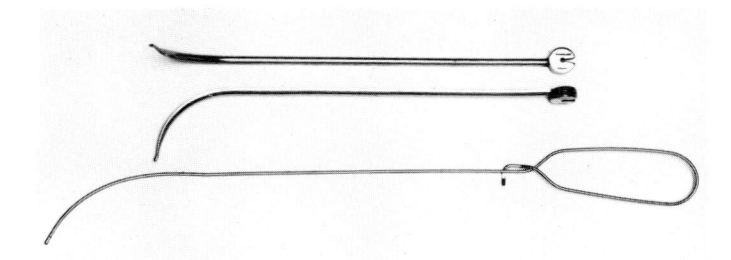

Fig.220 Wire and Maryfield catheter introducer

through a relatively bloodless field. In order to expose the renal sinus, Gill-Vernet designed special retractors for this purpose. These hand-held retractors are of graduated size. The retracting end is concave and lipped to follow the anatomical curve of the sinus.

For extraction of stones from the pelvis and calyces, renal stone extracting forceps are required. The most commonly used patterns are Turner–Warwick, Randall and Ward. These have several features in common. The ends of the jaws are gently curved and each jaw has a circular or oval fenestration which matches the opposite side. This fenestration serves to accommodate the stone within the jaws of the instrument, taking account of the confined space of the renal pelvis. Without the fenestrations the jaws would be opened by a distance equal to the size of the stone and this would hamper the stone removal within the confine of the renal pelvis. Some jaws, such as those of the Randall and Ward forceps, have serrations to improve grip on the stone.

All renal stone forceps are supplied in sets with curves ranging from slight to a deep retro. Because of the relatively small jaw size, the Turner–Warwick forceps are more suitable for nephrolithotomy.

Gil-Vernet, J.M. (1978) Pyelolithotomy in operative surgery. In: *Urology*, 3rd edn. (ed. Williams, D.J.). Butterworth, London

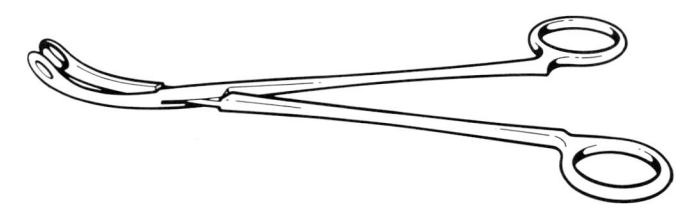

Fig.221 Turner Warwick calculus forceps (Downs)

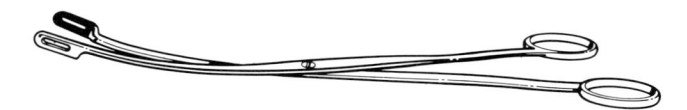

Fig.222 Rendall renal calculus forceps (Downs)

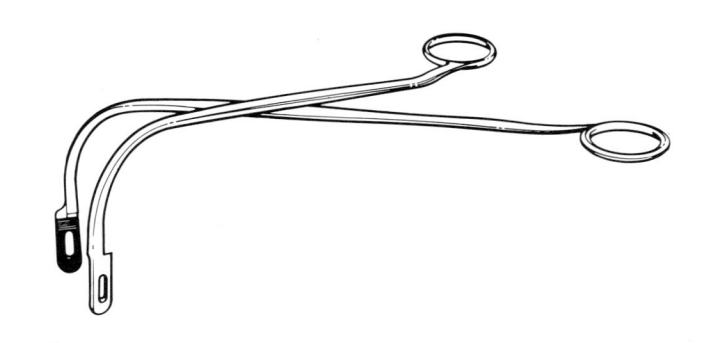

Fig.223 Rendall renal calculus forceps (Downs)

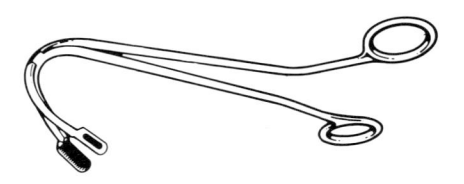

Fig.224 Rendall renal calculus forceps (Downs)

11.7 Prostatectomy instruments

Although the technique of trans-urethral resection of prostate has many advantages over transvesical or retropubic prostatectomy, the latter technique is here to stay, especially for large prostatic adenomas. Transvesical prostatectomy was first described by McGill in 1887 and is now rarely used. It is particularly suitable when there is a coexisting bladder pathology, such as a stone or bladder diverticulum. It is not suitable for small fibrous prostates, carcinoma, or bladder neck obstruction due to a fibrous bar.

Two instruments are essential for this operation: a bladder retractor and a boomerang needle.

The Millin pattern is most commonly used, although Harris's instruments preceded these. The retractor's two lateral blades serve to retract the abdominal wound as well as the cystotomy incision, while bringing the vault of the bladder up to skin level. A posterior blade improves exposure of the trigone and bladder neck. The main difficulty in transvesical prostatectomy is haemostasis within the prostatic cavity.

Harris's needle and needle holder is a modification of Young's boomerang needle and is used mainly to facilitate haemostasis, especially from urethral branches of prostatic artery. It is a strong trochar needle whose tip moves in a circle of about 100°. This is achieved by a spring-loaded pushrod. When a cylinder in the proximal end of the handle is pushed, the rod transmits the movement to the needle, which rotates around a transverse rod. The rod pushes the base of the needle, thus imparting a circular motion. The suture is hooked over the needle notch by means of angular ligature-carrying forceps originally designed by Harris. The ligature is placed across one of the double jaws and held by the

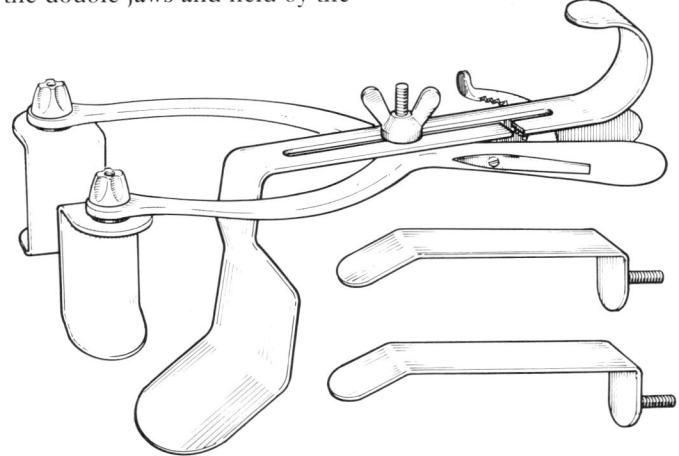

Fig.225 Millin retropubic retractor (Downs)

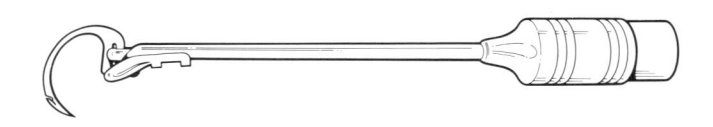

Fig.226 Millin boomerang needle holder (Downs)

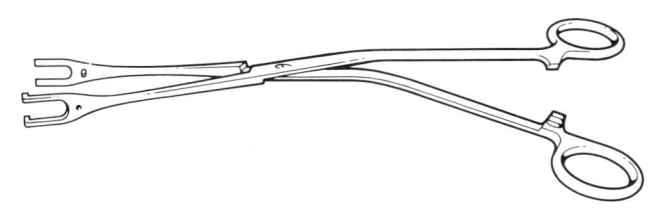

Fig.227 Millin ligature carrying forceps (Downs)

opposing jaw. The ligature lying in the jaw gap is then hooked over the needle notch and the grip released. By releasing the pressure on the boomerang needle handle, the needle moves back to its neutral position drawing the ligature with it.

Millin's retropubic prostatectomy obviates the need for cystotomy and provides good access to the prostatic bed. Again, good access is a must and Millin's retractor serves to retract the abdominal wound as well as pressing the empty bladder down by means of a third, Z-shaped blade. This blade not only retracts the bladder but also helps to define the bladder neck.

Bleeding from the edges of the prostatic capsule can be controlled by angular vulsellum forceps or Millin's prostatic capsule forceps. To improve exposure of the bladder neck during its resection and for haemostasis a Millin's bladder neck retractor is invaluable. This is a steel spring-loaded wire retractor whose ends are approximated by pressing the handle wires together; when released they spring apart.

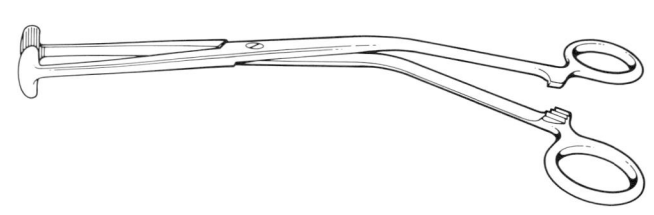

Fig.228 Millin prostatic capsule forceps (Downs)

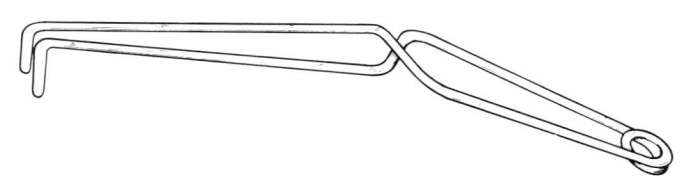

Fig.229 Millin bladder neck spreader (Downs)

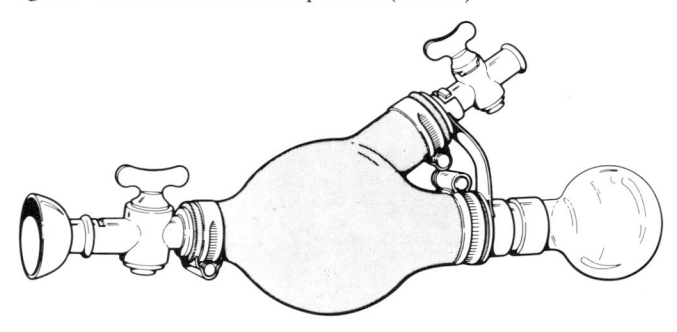

Fig.230 Bigelow evacuator (Downs)

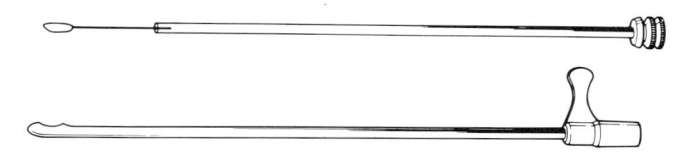

Fig.231 Metal catheter for Bigelow evacuator (Downs)

McGill, A.G. (1887) Suprapubic prostatectomy. *British Medical Journal*, 1887, **2**, 1104.

Feyer, P.J. (1900) A new method of performing prostatectomy. *Lancet*, 1900, **1**, 774.

Harris, S.H. (1929) Suprapubic prostatectomy with closure. *British Journal of Urology*, **1**, 285.

Macky, W. (1972) Transvesical prostatectomy. In: *Operative Surgery* (ed. Williams, I.D.), p. 243. Butterworths, London.

11.8 Bladder evacuator

The bladder evacuator was originally developed by Bigelow for washout of crushed bladder stone. The function of the evacuator is to swirl around the contents of the bladder before they are washed out. The Bigelow evacuator was connected to a metal cannula, now replaced with a resectoscope sheath.

The evacuator consists of a rubber bulb attached to a glass chamber and an attachment adaptor. The Bigelow evacuator has one single glass chamber attached below the rubber bulb.

The Ellik evacuator is a considerable improvement over Bigelow's, as it has two glass chambers, one above the other, with the bulb attached to the side of the upper chamber. Thus the bladder contents are first evacuated into the top chamber, which is subjected to swirling current, and then sink under gravity into the lower chamber. The Ellik evacuator is considerably lighter and less cumbersome, and is easier to sterlise.

Evacuation should be done gently as bladder perforation can occur. The evacuator must be filled completely with irrigating fluid. The presence of air, especially after transurethral resection, can produce air embolism.

Bigelow, H.J. (1879) Lithotrity by a single operation. *Boston Medical and Surgical Journal*, **98**, 259, 291.
Blandy, J. (1976) Stones and foreign bodies in the bladder. In: *Urology II* (ed. Blandy, J.), pp. 753-773. Blackwell Scientific Publications, Oxford.

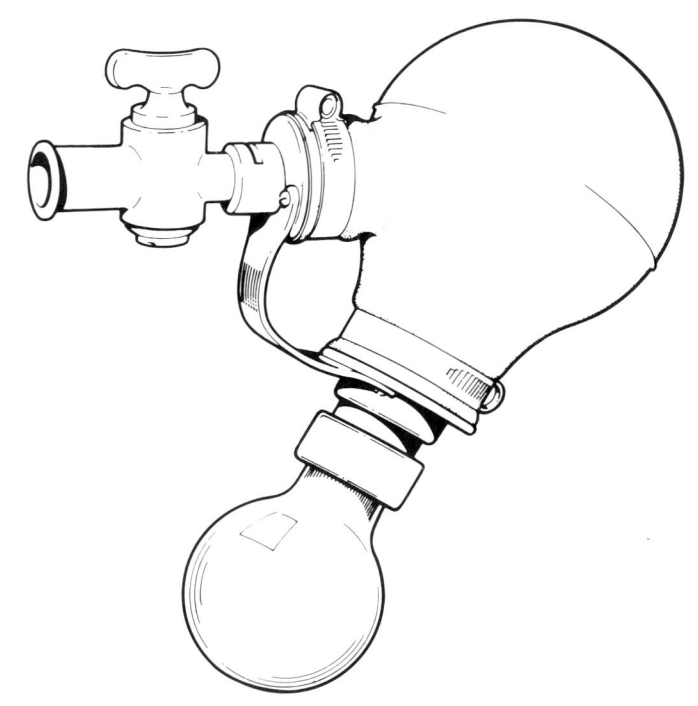

Fig.232 Freyer evacuator (Downs)

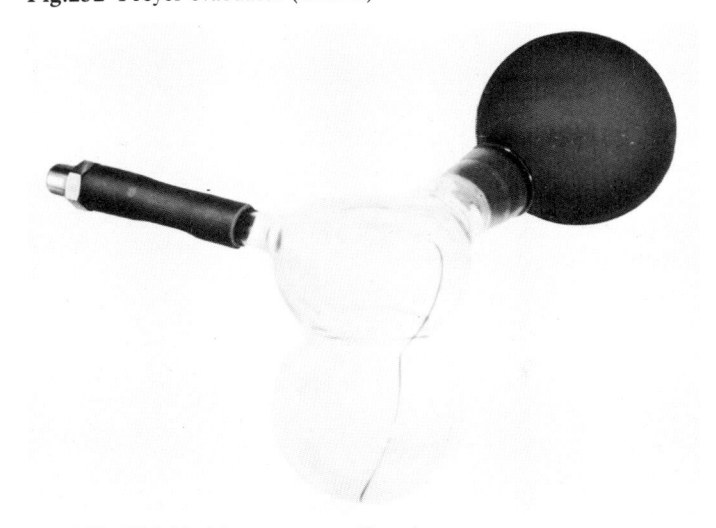

Fig.233 Ellik bladder evacuator (Storz)

11.9 Ureteric basket stone extractors

The introduction of basket ureteric extractors for ureteric stones was a logical extension of attempts at endoscopic stone extraction. In 1925, Council described a wire basket consisting of six flexible wires which were arranged side by side in the form of a spindle. The proximal end of the basket was attached to a short filiform bougie. The spindle was expanded by a central wire, which caused the approximation of the proximal and distal ends of the wire basket. The ureter was usually dilated before the passage of the instrument.

The Dormia extractor consists of a ureteric catheter (5 Ch) with a flexible wire rod within its lumen. The proximal end of the catheter has a screw mounting which allows control of the position of the wire. The distal end contains the spiral basket, consisting of four or more stainless steel wires, twisted to form a helical bobbin spindle. The end of the spindle has a cap which is of the same calibre as the introducing catheter. With the rod pulled down, the basket is contained entirely within the catheter. When the rod is pushed upwards the basket wires expand due to their elasticity and emerge as the spiral basket.

The new Dormia dislodger has a spiral cage made up of six wires, three running in one direction and the other three in the opposite direction. This arrangement has several advantages over the earlier four-wire design; there is no longer the risk of ureteric rotation during catheter withdrawal and the extraction of stones is more precise because of the increased density of the basket.

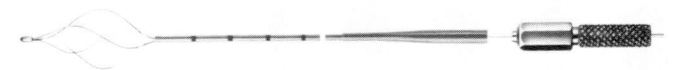

The Dormia extractor should not be used on stones larger than 5 mm, more than 5 cm from the ureteric orifice, in a hydroureter, in periureteritis or if previous manipulation has been carried out recently. The complications include ureteric wall perforation or even avulsion. Should the extractor become lodged with the stone *in situ* it is best to leave the catheter in place and wait for it to pass spontaneously.

Fig.234 Dormia stone dislodger (Storz)

Council, W.A. (1925) New ureteral stone extractor and dilation. *Journal of the American Medical Association*, **86**, 1907.
Council, W.A. (1945) The treatment of ureteral calculi: report of 504 cases in which Council stone extractor and dilator was used. *Journal of Urology*, **53**, 534.
Dormia, F. and Bassi, R. (1961) Radiological collaboration in the endoscopic removal of ureteric stone with the Dormia extractor. *Urologia*, **28**, 355.

11.10 Percutaneous pyelolithotomy

Until very recently, direct visualisation of intrarenal drainage system and pelvis was possible only in open surgery.

Percutaneous nephrostomy was first described in 1955 by Goodwin and it was not until 1976 that Fernström and Johansson described percutaneous removal of renal stones via a pre-existing nephrostomy. However, the limiting factor in this procedure was the size of the stone, which could not exceed the size of the nephrostomy channel.

This problem has been overcome by the introduction of stone disintegration instruments under direct vision. This new technique, together with extracorporeal shock wave lithotripsy has opened new horizons in the treatment of renal calculi and will undoubtedly soon replace the direct surgical approach.

Percutaneous nephrostomy can be performed under local or general anaesthesia. The patient is positioned on an X-ray table in the prone position. The puncture site, which usually lies in the posterior axillary line between the twelfth rib and the iliac crest, is determined by fluoroscopy. This approach is used for transparenchymal access, thus avoiding the larger renal vessels. A more medial approach into a dilated collecting system will cause the system to collapse, thus making further dilatation difficult if not impossible. Either the lower or the middle calyceal system is chosen depending on the position of the stone.

The chosen calyx is punctured with a fine needle and a J guide wire is inserted under screening. The track is dilated up to 7 FG with a catheter introducer set. Further dilatation up to 24 FG is carried out with a telescopic dilatation set.

Under local anaesthesia the dilatation is performed on two or three sessions over a period of several days. A nephrostomy tube is left *in situ* between dilatations. The 27 FG nephroscope sheath is inserted into the tract at the final stage of dilatation. The working channel of the rigid nephroscope accepts baskets, forceps, loops and the ultrasound probe.

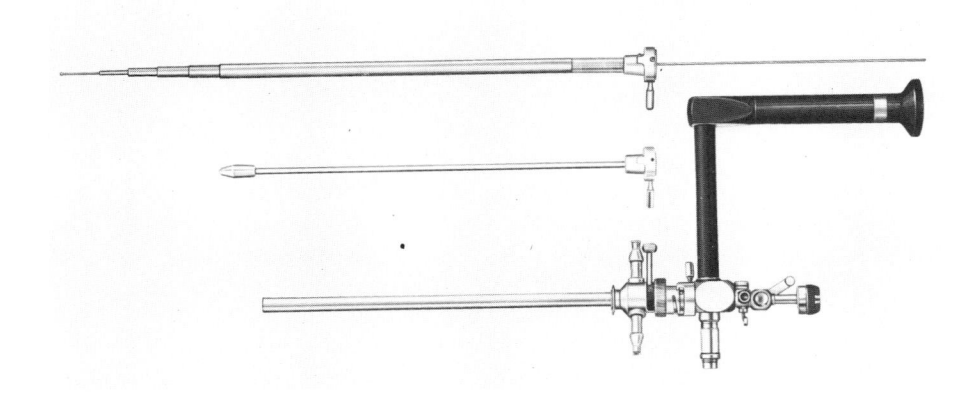

Fig.235 Storz percutaneous nephroscope and telescopic dilators

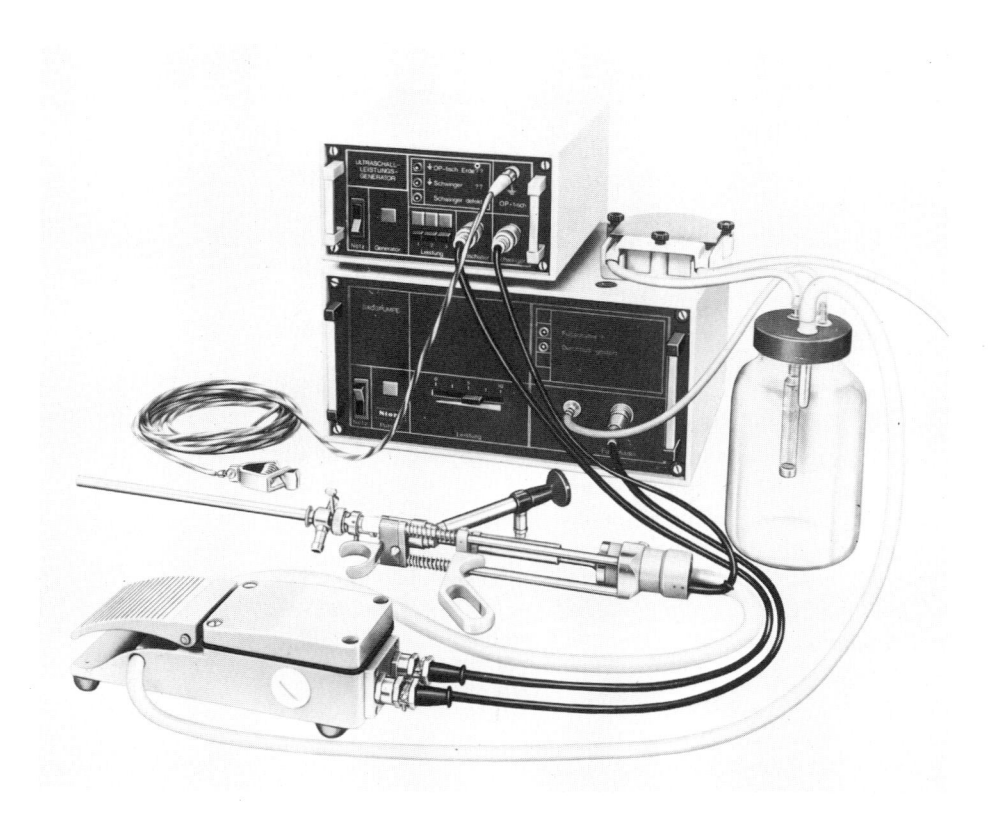

Fig.236 Storz percutaneous lithotripsy ultrasound assembly

Renal stones can be removed by several methods. Chemolysis is successful only in a small percentage of stones, mainly those composed of uric acid, cystine or struvite—apatite.

This technique requires two nephrostomy tubes, one for inflow and the other for outflow. It may take more than 30 daily treatments to dissolve stones.

Mechanical stone removal is limited by the size of the stone. Providing the stone is smaller than the sheath of the scope, it can be extracted with forceps or Dormia basket.

Large stones can be broken up with an ultrasound probe and the fragments removed in the same way as the smaller stones. The fine grit and dust is sucked out through the central channel of the ultrasound probe.

Finally, the complete stone clearance is confirmed by X-rays, and contrast dye introduced into the collecting system confirms free flow into the bladder. After the procedure the nephrostomy tract dries up within several days providing no obstruction to outflow is present.

Goodwin, W.E., Casey, W.C. and Woolf, W. (1965) Percutaneous trocar (needle) nephrostomy in hydronephrosis. *Journal of the American Medical Association,* **157**, 891.

Fernström, I. and Johansson, B. (1976) Percutaneous pyelolithotomy. A new extraction technique. *Scandinavian Journal of Urology and Nephrology,* **10**, 257.

Alken, R., Hutscheinreiter, G. and Günther, R. (1982) Percutaneous kidney stone removal. *European Urology,* **8**, 304-311.

Chapter 12   Orthopaedics

12.1 Bone instruments
12.2 Bone fixation
12.3 Limb traction
12.4 Plaster and plaster instruments

12.1 Bone instruments

Orthopaedic surgery deals mostly with bones, and orthopaedic tools are designed to cut, trim or manipulate them.

The simplest way of cutting bone is with a saw. Bone hand-saws were originally designed for amputation. Fergusson's saw is characterised by a rigid back which reinforces the thin blade attached to the handle. This rigid back is attached to the handle by a screw and can be lifted out should it be in the way during sawing, or for cleaning. It is sometimes called the standard amputation saw for the British Army. Adam's saw was described in 1870 and was designed for subcutaneous division of the femoral neck. The short, narrow blade is integral with a long arm and handle. The tip of the blade is blunt to prevent injury during blind sawing. Butcher, an Irish surgeon, designed a considerably heavier instrument characterised by its massive frame and a long, narrow blade which is stretched by a nut-and-screw mechanism on the frame. The blades are interchangable. Because of its size this saw is more suitable for above-knee amputations. Power saws have virtually replaced hand saws in modern orthopaedic practice. Most are of the oscillating type developed by Stryker and are powered by air, gas or

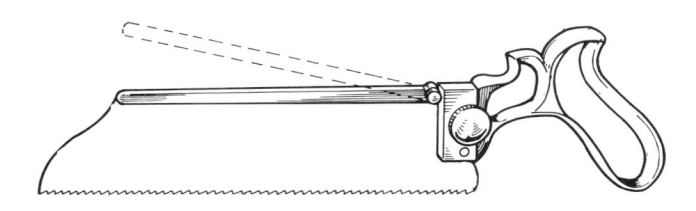

Fig.237 Fergusson amputation saw (Downs)

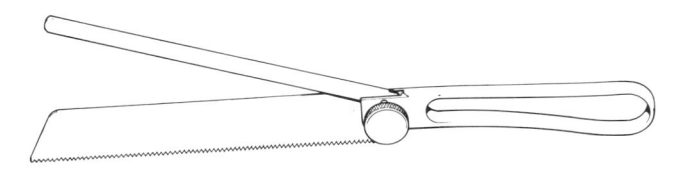

Fig.238 Army regulation amputation saw (Downs)

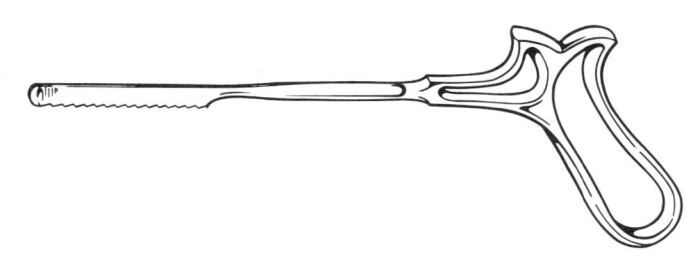

Fig.239 Adams-Jones saw (Downs)

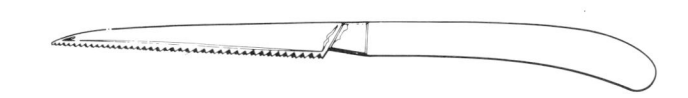

Fig.240 Finger saw

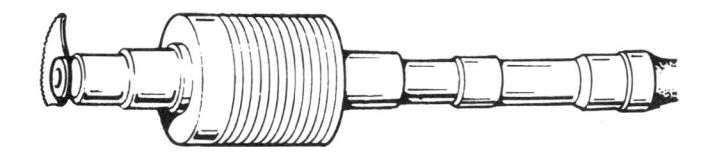

Fig.241 Stryker oscillating saw (Downs)

electricity. The saw oscillates through a small arc at a frequency of 25 000 – 30 000 oscillations per minute. Soft tissues adjacent to the bone are not cut unless they lie between the blade and the bone.

The orthopaedic chisel is a wedge-like instrument where the cutting edge has a straight side and tapering side. The osteotome was introduced into surgery in 1879 by William McEwan, who pointed out the disadvantages of a chisel for cutting into bone. It has a straight edge, the sides of which taper equally. An osteotome passes readily and accurately into bone and can be easily withdrawn. The handle of McEwan's osteotome is octagonal for better grip.

Bone gouges are used to remove small pieces of bone, as in abscess deroofing, and for cutting grooves. The cutting surface is curved from side to side. After cutting a semicircular segment of bone the blade has the tendency to leave the bone, instead of cutting further. It also leaves the cut surface smooth, which is important as it minimises the danger of bone sepsis.

A mallet is essentially a hammer with a large head. They are either all metal, wooden or plastic. Some metal mallets have lead-filled heads but these rapidly lose shape. Metal mallets with a plastic-covered striking surface are less noisy and cushion the shock on instrument handles.

Periosteal elevators and rougines are described elsewhere.

A file is a steel instrument roughened for shaping, and a rasp is a

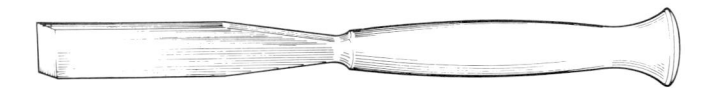

Fig.242 Smith-Petersen chisel (Downs)

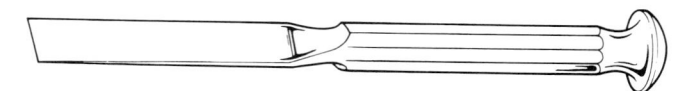

Fig.243 McEwan osteotome (Downs)

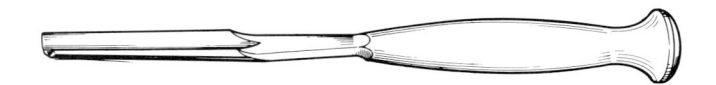

Fig.244 Smith-Petersen gouge (Downs)

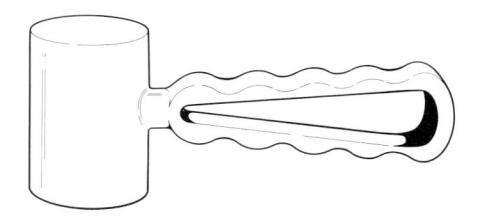

Fig.245 Heath mallet (Downs)

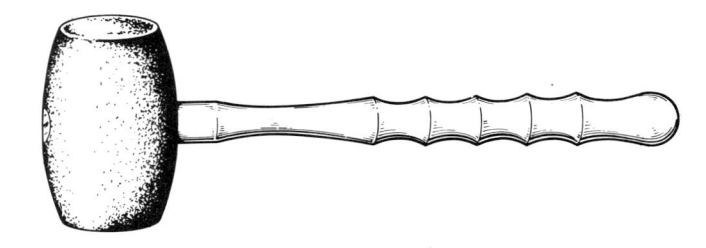

Fig.246 Rubber-headed mallet (Downs)

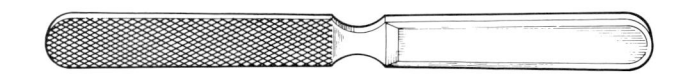

Fig.247 Bone file and rasp (Downs)

coarse file having separate teeth. They are both used for smoothing or shaping bone surfaces and edges.

Bone-cutting forceps are like wire-cutters. For cutting through large bones they have double-action joints. Liston's forceps are probably the best known and are very versatile.

Bone-holding forceps are designed for manipulation of bone ends and fragments. They have long handles for better leverage and small jaws which make contact at their tips. The gripping surface of the jaws has teeth or serrations for better grip with minimal bruising to the bone. Hey Groves's bone-holding forceps are designed for grasping large, circular bones, such as the femur. The jaws have transverse serrations and grip on the handles can be maintained by means of a fly nut. Some forceps employ a ratchet mechanism instead.

12.2 Bone fixation

The alternative to splinting and traction for the treatment of fractures is external or internal fixation. External bone fixation is not a new technique and has been practised since the beginning of this century. It is used most commonly to stabilise fractures of long bones, especially if these are compound or comminuted. Its main advantages over the traditional forms of splinting are that: it provides stable immobilisation of the fracture without immobilising the proximal and distal joints; it provides direct access to the wound; and it allows early mobilisation

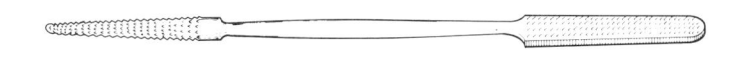

Fig.248 Putti rasp

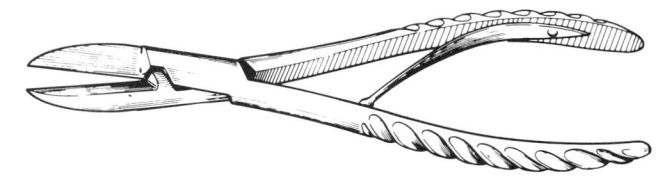

Fig.249 Liston bone-cutting forceps

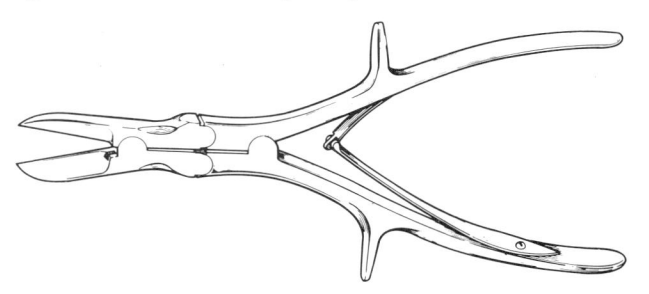

Fig.250 Horsley Liston bone-cutting forceps (Downs)

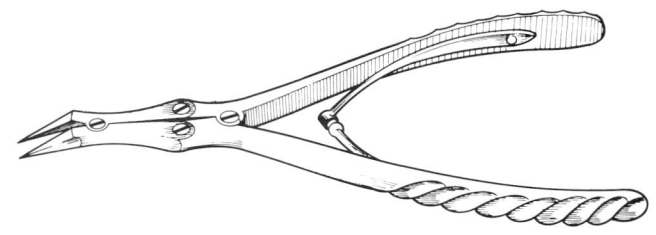

Fig.251 McIndoe bone-cutting forceps (Downs)

Fig.252 Hey Groves bone-holding forceps (Downs)

of the patient. This technique is also used in pelvic diastasis, osteotomies and arthrodeses.

There are two main types of external fixation: frames and single bars. The Hoffman frame is the most widely used system and is also very reliable. It consists of interlocking rods which can be extended or retracted, and to these the ends of pins are attached. The pins are inserted proximal and distal to the fracture. The rod joints then allow the bone ends to be compressed or distracted and aligned, as required.

The single rod system is similar in principle but these appliances are much simpler and cheaper. The pins are inserted into the cortex of the bone on either side of the fracture and are attached to the main bar by small plates. Again, the fracture can be compressed or distracted by means of a control screw.

Internal fixation is a means of immobilisation by devices implanted in the vicinity of the fracture. This technique is mainly indicated when long-term immobilisation in bed is undesirable, when it is necessary to restore contour of joints involved in the fracture, in patients with multiple injuries, and as a treatment for fracture non-union. Internal fixation can be achieved with medullary nails, plates, nail plates, screws or wires.

Medullary nails are particularly suitable for long bones, such as the femur or humerus. Strong nails, such as Rush's, may be inserted through the fracture by driving it through the proximal segment first and then down across the fracture. Alternatively, they may be inserted percutaneously. Kirschner wires are suitable for small bones in the hands and feet.

Screws are used either alone to hold pieces of bone together, or to hold plates onto bones. There are two types of screws used for fractures: machine and ASIF screws. Machine screws are threaded along their whole length and may be self-tapping or may require threads to be cut prior to their insertion. The size of the drilled hole is critical. ASIF screws were designed for the technique of osteosynthesis by the ASIF group. They have more horizontal threads and are not self-tapping. The drill hole must be tapped with a tapper before the screws are inserted. There are many different designs for cortical, cancellous and malleolar bones, as well as for screwing small fragments of bone. Plates and screws are used for internal fixation of diaphyseal fractures. The plates must be strong and malleable to allow for adjustment to the contour of the bone. The screws must be of the same alloy as the plate to prevent corrosion. There are three main designs of straight ASIF plates currently in use. The regular type has round screw holes and is applied under compression using a plate compressioner. The dynamic compression plate has screw holes which utilise the spherical gliding principle. As the screw is tightened its head is guided by the contours of the hole so that it glides towards the centre of the plate, resulting in the bone fragments being displaced in the same direction, that is towards the fracture. The semitubular plates are thin and semicircular in cross section. The screw holes are oval. As the screw heads engage the edges of the screw holes, compression of the fracture ends results. These plates are used mainly for subcutaneous bones where rigidity is not an important factor. Loops of wire can be used for holding fragments of both together, in conjunction with other methods of internal fixation. This technique is called cerclage.

Batten, R.L. (1979) General techniques of internal fixation of fractures. In: *Operative Surgery*, 3rd edn. (ed. Rob, C. & Smith, R.), pp. 55-75, Butterworth, London.

Müller, M.E., Allgöwer, M. and Willenegger, H. (1970) *Manual of Internal Fixation*. Springer-Verlag, Berlin.

12.3 Limb traction

Traction is designed to counteract the deforming forces which act on a fractured bone, as well as to control the movement that takes place between fracture surfaces. It can be applied to the skin or the skeleton. In order to prevent the body from being pulled in the direction of the traction force a countertraction has to be applied. The weight of the body itself provides a degree of countertraction. When countertraction is applied through a mechanical appliance the arrangement is called fixed traction.

Skin traction has application mainly in children and where the traction force required to maintain reduction is not great. The maximum skin traction weight is 7 kg. The traction force is applied to a large area of skin by means of an adhesive or non-adhesive strapping. The absolute contraindication to this form of traction is impaired circulation and wounds and abrasions of the skin under traction. Complications of skin traction are limited to allergic reactions to adhesive, pressure sores and nerve palsies due to pressure.

Skeletal traction is virtually limited to fractures of the lower limb and cervical spine (section 14.5). The traction force is applied to the skeleton via a pin or screw driven through the bone.

The Steinmann pin is a rigid stainless steel rod, 4–6 mm in diameter. The pin is mounted on an introducer and the sharp point is driven through the skin and bone until it appears through the opposite side. A stirrup is fitted to each end of the pin and guards are attached to prevent accidental injury.

The Denham pin differs from Steinmann's in that it has a length of thread on the shaft which engages in the bony cortex. The thread prevents the pin from sliding.

Kirschner wire is a thin rod of stainless steel which must be stretched in a special stirrup before traction is applied. It is unsuitable for heavy traction, as it easily cuts through the bone, and is therefore more suitable for upper limb traction.

In special circumstances, for instance in central fracture-dislocations of the hip, lateral traction may be required in addition to axial traction. This can be achieved by inserting a coarse-threaded screw into the femoral neck. A length of stainless steel wire is attached to it and brought out through the skin incision.

The main complications of skeletal traction are pin loosening, infection, joint stiffness and bone splintering during pin insertion. Should the traction force be too great, the fracture ends may become sufficiently distracted to cause delayed union.

Stewart, J.D.M. (1979) External fixation of fractures. In: *Operative Surgery*, 3rd edn. (ed. Rob. C. and Smith, R.), pp. 76-92. Butterworth, London.

12.3 Plaster and plaster instruments

Fracture splinting has been practised for several thousand years. Prior to the introduction of plaster of Paris various materials were used for this purpose. As recently as World War I, the British Army used bamboo splints as a standard issue in India. Plaster of Paris, the hydrate of calcium sulphate, has been known since ancient times, although it was introduced for the treatment of fractures in the early nineteenth century. Its name derives from a large mine north of Paris where it was produced.

Initially the limb was dipped into a tub containing plaster. In the mid nineteenth century, plaster bandages were introduced. The modern plaster of Paris is the hemihydrate, which dissolves in water and, when dry, crystallises and becomes solid.

A large number of new materials have been introduced as alternatives to plaster of Paris. Their advantages and disadvantages, as well as indications for use, will not be discussed. They include epoxy resins, thermoplastics and fibreglass. Baycast (Bayer) is a conventional bandage impregnated with polyurethane resin, which is immersed in water prior to application. It sets in five minutes and full weight can be applied in 30 minutes. The material is light, water resistant and radiolucent. It is also easy to remove. Zoroc (Johnson & Johnson) and Cellamin (Lohmann) combine plaster with resin. The resin makes the cast stronger, lighter and water resistant. Hexcelite is a thermoplastic polymer with an inorganic filler which is applied to a bandage. The bandage is softened by immersion in hot water, and applied. It sets in three minutes and full weight bearing can be permitted in 15 minutes. The cast is light, strong and waterproof. Lightcast (3M Company) is an example of a fibreglass cast. The bandage, made of porous fibreglass, is impregnated with photosensitive resin which is activated by ultraviolet light and sets in three minutes.

A variety of instruments have been designed for plaster removal. The plaster knife is no longer used because of its inherent dangers. Plaster shears are safer and much more popular. They are essentially heavy-duty scissors with angled blades. The inner blade is longer and has a flat, blunt tip to prevent injury and to guide the instrument along the inner surface of the cast. The heavy-duty plaster shears are essentially wire-cutters with long handles. The oscillating saw, described in section 12.1, is not without hazard and should be used with care over bony prominences and where padding is deficient or thin. An alternative method of cutting plaster is to bury a Gigli saw under the cast and to saw through it when the cast is ready to be removed. This principle has recently been reintroduced in the form of the Arthrodax orthopaedic cast wire. This is a double strand of cabled wire which is attached to a plastic button. The wire is buried under the cast, which can be broken by winding the free wire ends on to a winding bar with a ratchet handle.

Monro, J.K. (1935) The history of plaster of Paris in the treatment of fractures. *British Journal of Surgery*, **23**, 257.

Hunt, D.M. (1980) New materials for the immobilization of fractures. *British Journal of Hospital Medicine*, September 1980, 273-275.

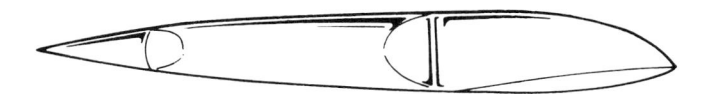

Fig.253 Esmarch plaster of Paris knife (Downs)

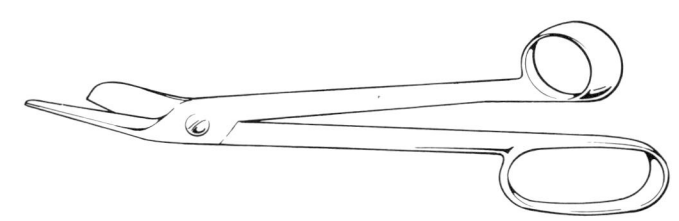

Fig.254 Guy plaster shears (Downs)

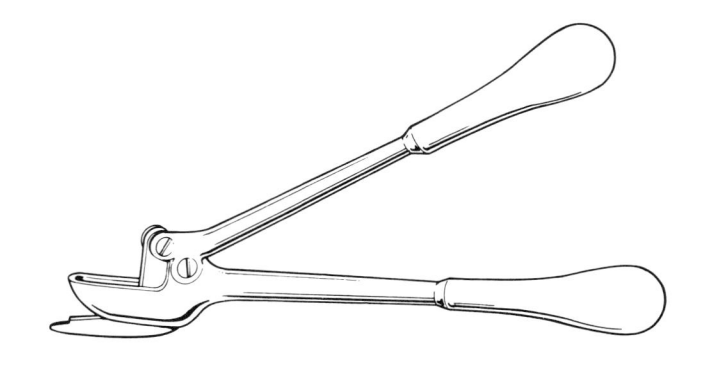

Fig.255 Lorenz plaster shears (Downs)

Chapter 13 Vascular and Thoracic Surgery

13.1 Vein strippers
13.2 Cardiovascular forceps, scissors and clamps
13.3 Endarterectomy instruments
13.4 Aneurysm and pedicle needles
13.5 Amputation instruments
13.6 Thoracic instruments
13.7 Sternum-splitting instruments
13.8 Rib raspatories (rougine)
13.9 Rib shears
13.10 Rib retractors and approximators
13.11 Oesophageal dilators

13.1 Vein strippers

Recently there has been a swing by surgeons away from long and short saphenous vein stripping for varicose veins. This is mainly because it has been realised that saphenous veins are not always connected with lower limb varicosities and consequently stripping may not be curative.

Equally, the long saphenous vein has proved useful in femoro-popliteal and coronary bypass and it is therefore in the patient's interest to preserve this vein should the need for it arise.

Mayo originally designed a ring vein stripper which was passed on the outside of veins. Myers' vein stripper, or one of its many modifications, is passed intraluminally. It consists of a coiled spring with a wire core approximately 90 cms long. One end has a blunt tip and the other is fitted with an acorn-shaped head of various sizes.

Some strippers have a detachable handle which is attached to the blunt olivary tip of the stripper. Modern disposable strippers have the advantage of being pre-sterilised and have a smooth outer plastic casing. They also may have an offset coiled end to help in negotiating difficult segments of the vein.

The leading olivary-tipped end of the stripper is passed along the lumen of the vein, usually in the proximal direction, to avoid venous valves and deviation into the main tributaries. It is then withdrawn through the divided proximal end of the vein. The distal end of the vein is divided and ligature tied around the stripper just proximal to the acorn-shaped head. By pulling the end of the stripper proximally, the vein is avulsed.

Rivlin, S. (1951) *Treatment of Varicose Veins and their Complications*. Heinemann, London.

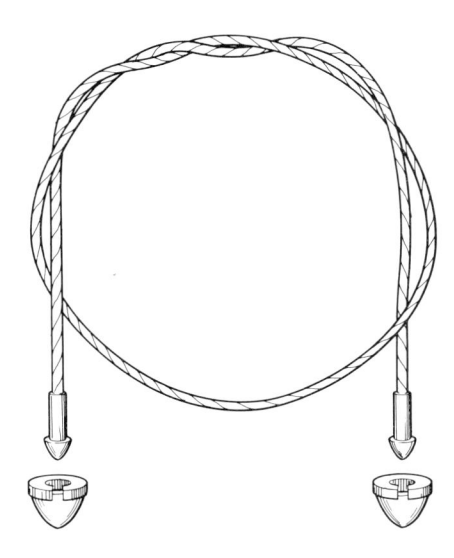

Fig.256 Graves & Blower varicose stripper (Downs)

Rivlin, S. (1975) The surgical care of primary varicose veins. *British Journal of Surgery*, **62**, 913-917.

13.2 Cardiovascular forceps, scissors and clamps

Blood vessels have to be handled gently and there is no place for toothed dissecting forceps. Cardiovascular forceps must be able to grip tissues firmly and safely and yet without injury. For that reason they have multiple fine teeth, or serrations, that interdigitate, allowing them to grip the vessel wall without crushing. The most well known examples are de Bakey's forceps.

Scissors should be fine and accurate. Pott's scissors are angled and are used specifically for incising or excising the vessel wall.

Two types of clamp are used. The bulldog clamp is used for small blood vessels. The Satinsky-type clamps are made in different shapes and sizes, to suit the size and accessibility of the vessel.

13.3 Endarterectomy instruments

Endarterectomy still has a place in vascular surgery. If it is limited to a short segment of the vessel then the atheroma can easily be shelled out using a Watson Cheyne probe and dissector. However, long segments of atheroma can only be removed with a loop stripper, first introduced by Cannon in 1955. The upper and lower

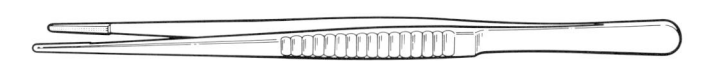

Fig.257 DeBakey tissue forceps (Downs)

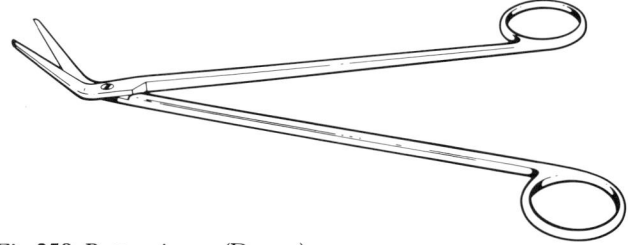

Fig.258 Potts scissors (Downs)

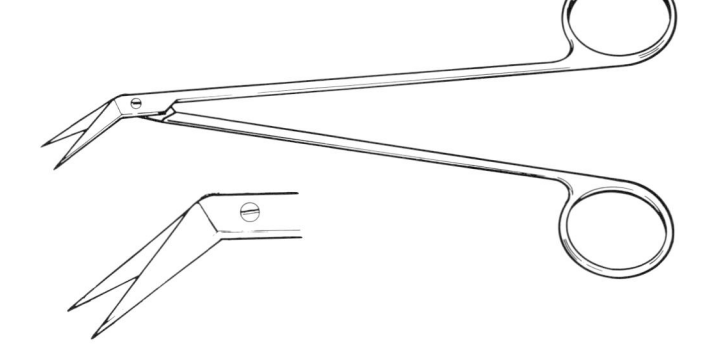

Fig.259 DeBakey scissors (Downs)

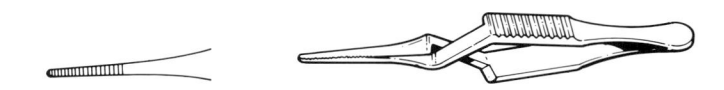

Fig.260 Mini bulldog clamp (Downs)

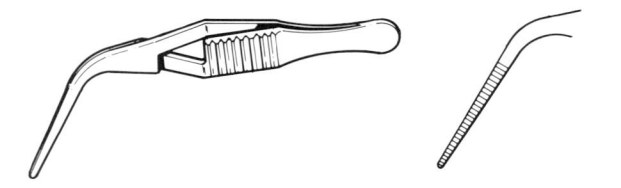

Fig.261 Curved mini bulldog clamp (Downs)

ends of atheroma are exposed through arteriotomy incisions and the atheroma shelled out and divided. The ring stripper of internal diameter corresponding to the that of the atheroma is passed over the atheromatous plug and gradually passed along the vessel, thus separating it from the vessel wall. The loop has a cutting edge.

Vollmar's ring strippers are blunt, and rings are obliquely inclined. They are particularly suitable for long atheromatous segments in medium-sized vessels.

Cannon, J.A. and Barker, W.F. (1955) Successful management of obstructive femoral arteriosclerosis by endarterectomy. *Surgery*, **38**, 48.

Vollmar, J., Trede, M., Lanbach, K. and Forrest, H. (1968) Principles of reconstructive procedures for chronic femoro-popliteal occlusions. Report on 546 operations. *Annals of Surgery*, **168**, 215.

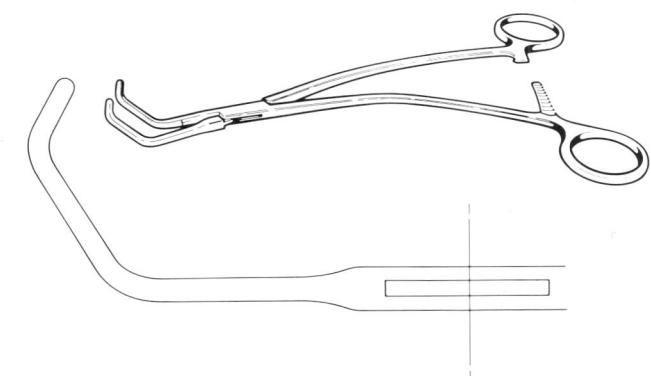

Fig.262 Satinski vena cava clamp (Downs)

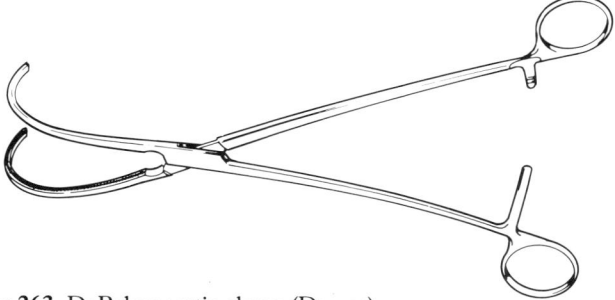

Fig.263 DeBakey aortic clamp (Downs)

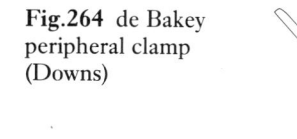

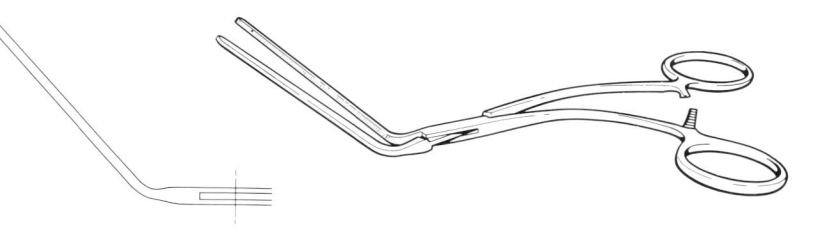

Fig.264 de Bakey peripheral clamp (Downs)

Fig.265 DeBakey aortic clamp (Downs)

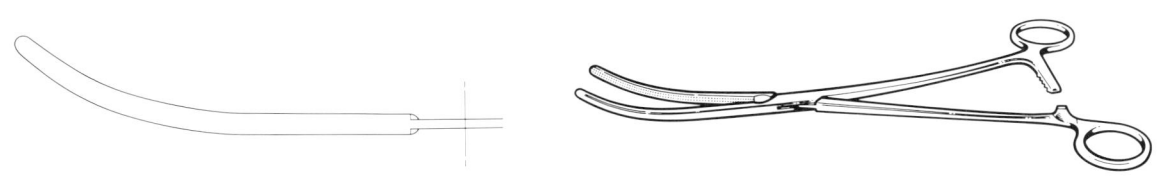

144 OPERATIVE INSTRUMENTS

Fig.266 Rumel forceps (Downs)

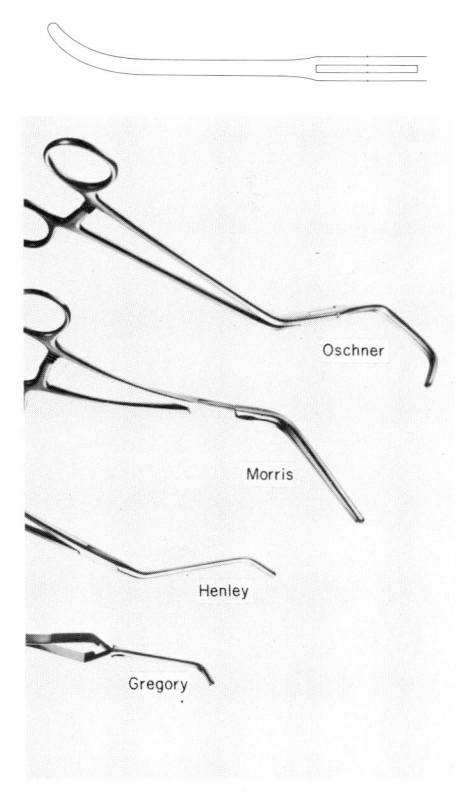

Fig.267 Vascular clamps (Codman)

13.4 Aneurysm and pedicle needles

Aneurysm needles are used for passing ligature round vessels and were originally used for ligature of aneurysms.

These needles are curved in one plane only, with the end blunt and flattened. The ligature is passed through an eye placed immediately

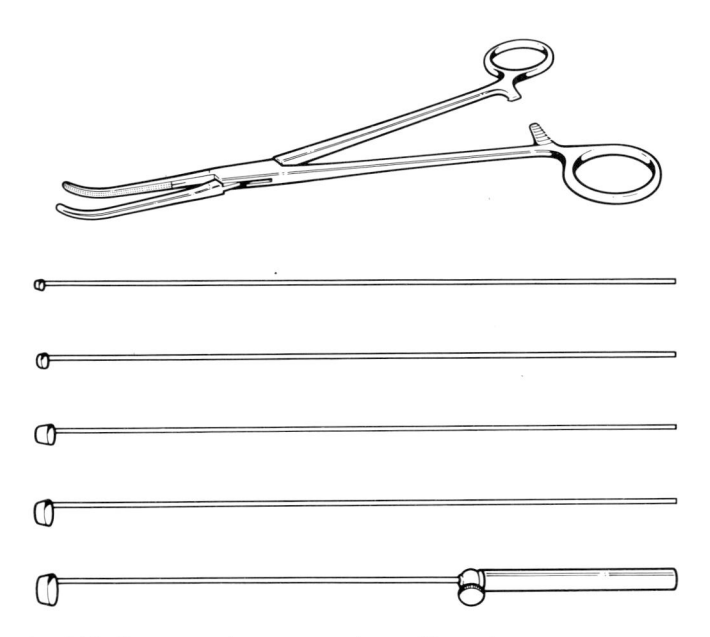

Fig.268 Cannon endarterectomy loops (Downs)

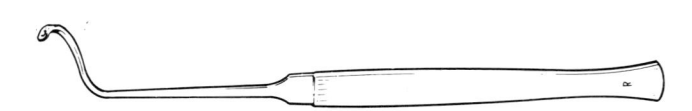

Fig.269 Dupuytren aneurysm needle (Downs)

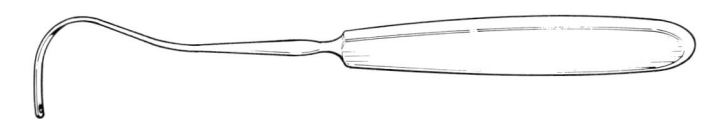

Fig.270 Joll aneurysm needle (Downs)

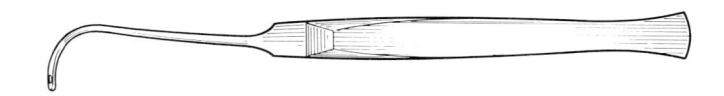

Fig.271 Syme aneurysm needle

behind the point of the needle. Best known are Dupuytren's and Syme's needles.

Pedicle needles are similar to aneurysm needles but they are tapered. They are used for transfixion of pedicles. Cleveland's pedicle needle consists of two thin, tapering blades operated by handles. The tip of one blade forms the needle tip and the other blade grasps the ligature.

Macewen's hernia needles are really aneurysm needles which are curved in two planes. They are now rarely used for hernia repair but can usefully be used as aneurysm needles.

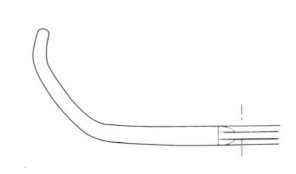

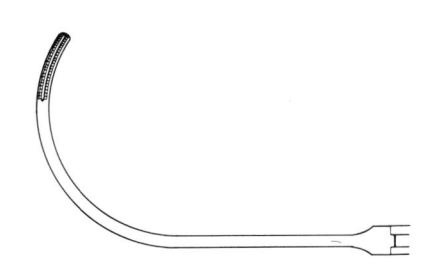

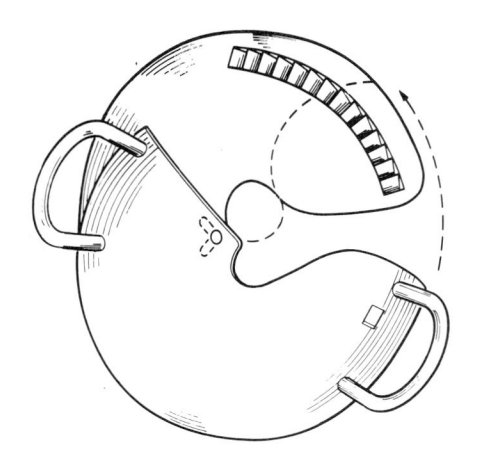

Fig.272 Blake amputation flap retractor (Downs)

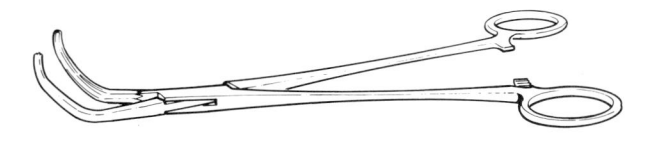

Fig.273 Price Thomas bronchus clamp (Downs)

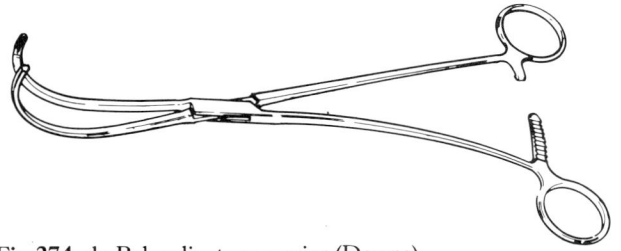

Fig.274 de Bakey ligature carrier (Downs)

13.5 Amputation instruments

Amputation, one of the oldest operations, is still performed, although perhaps with less speed and more attention to skin flaps than previously. Skin incision and skin flaps are made with a scalpel. Amputation knives are

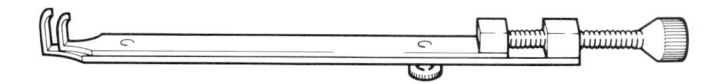

Fig.275 Blalock pulmonary artery clamp

suitable for dividing fascia and muscle. The vascular bundle is divided between artery forceps and ligated.

The periosteum is elevated with a rougine. The bone can be divided with a hand-held or mechanical saw. The most commonly used hand-held saws are Fergusson's and Butcher's (section 10.4).

Using a protector for thigh muscles, the cut end of bone is smoothed or bevelled with a file.

13.6 Thoracic instruments

Thoracic instruments are not much different from those for general surgery. The main difference is that they all have elongated handles.

Prior to the introduction of dissection technique in lobectomy, the hilum of the lung was controlled with a tourniquet. Bronchus clamps, such as Tudor-Edwards's, are curved, strong forceps whose jaws are longitudinally serrated and have interlocking multiple sharp teeth. Holme Sellors's bronchus clamp is of similar design except that it lacks interlocking teeth.

13.7 Sternum-splitting instruments

The chest can be opened either laterally by resecting one or two ribs or anteriorly by splitting the sternum.

The sternum can simply be cut longitudinally using a powered Stryker saw. Alternatively, having tunnelled under the sternum, a Gigli saw can be passed in and used to split the

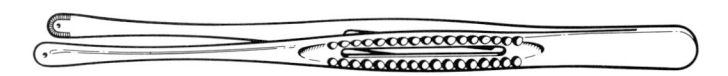

Fig.276 Mayo lung forceps (Downs)

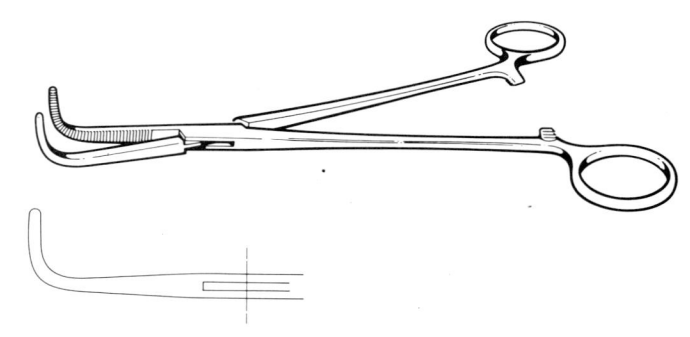

Fig.277 O'Shaughnessy artery forceps (Downs)

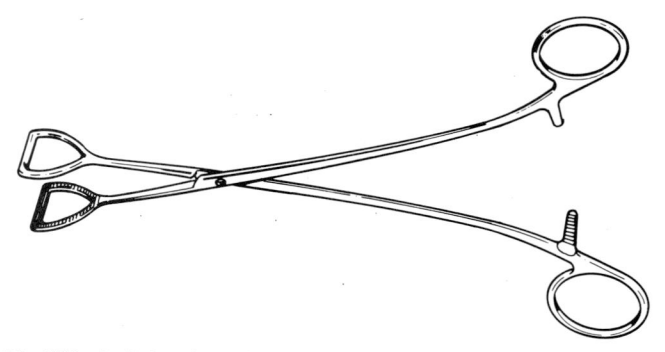

Fig.278 de Bakey lung forceps (Downs)

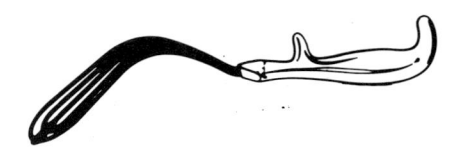

Fig.279 Allison lung retractor (Downs)

sternum. The Sauerbruch sternal splitter is a heavy and powerful instrument. The longer, fixed jaw is passed under and parallel to the sternum and by approximating the handles the mobile, smaller jaw shears through the bone making a longitudinal cut. The instrument is then moved further forward and the operation repeated.

13.8 Rib raspatories (rougine)

The importance of periosteal preservation in rib resection has long been known. Tools made to scrape and elevate the periosteum have been called by a variety of names: rougines, raspatories, bone scrapers or peristeal elevators.

Having exposed the rib, a longitudinal incision is made over its outer surface with a scalpel. The periosteum is stripped off the outer surface of the rib using Farabeuf's rougine, which is made with a straight, curved or fenestrated end. In effect it is a three-sided chisel.

When the outer surface of the rib is free of periosteum a Doyen raspatory, either left or right handed, is passed behind the rib, between it and the periosteum. It is then slid along the rib, usually in the anterior direction. It will strip off periosteum without injuring the bone.

13.9 Rib shears

A freed rib can be removed by using bone-cutting forceps such as Liston's.

Fig.280 Sauerbruch sternum cutter (Downs)

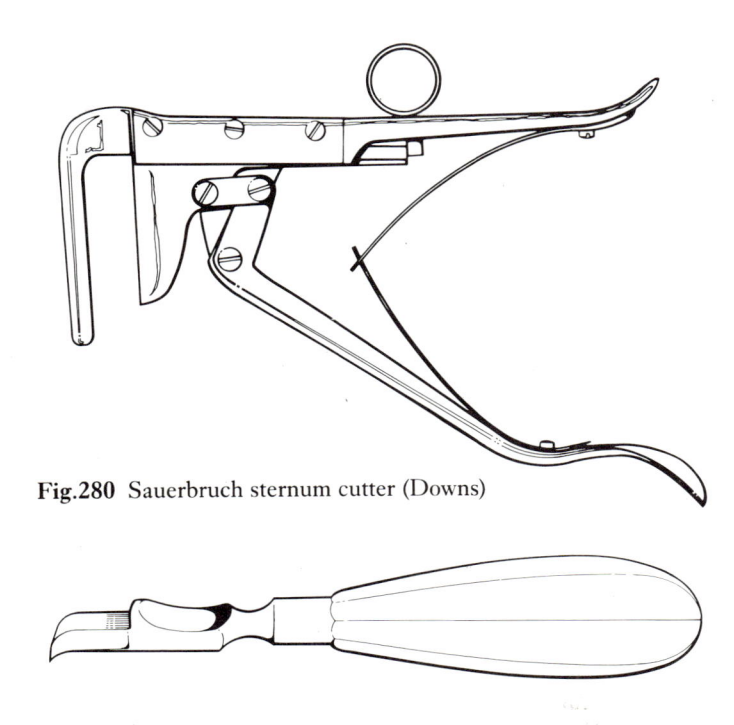

Fig.281 Farabeuf rougine (Downs)

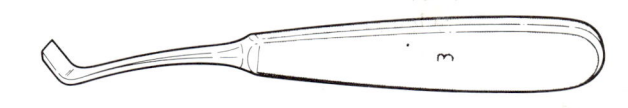

Fig.282 Semb rib raspatory (Downs)

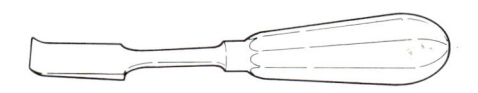

Fig.283 Tudor Edwards periosteal elevator (Downs)

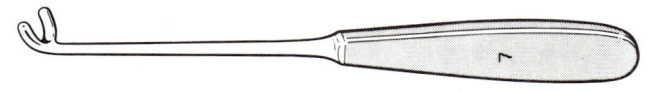

Fig.284 Semb rib raspatory (Downs)

148 OPERATIVE INSTRUMENTS

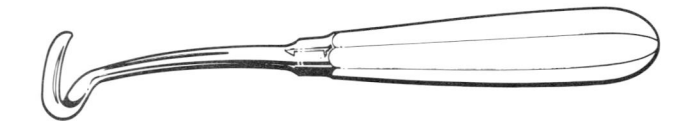

Fig.285 Doyen periosteal elevator (Downs)

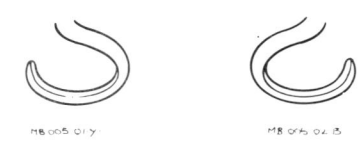

However, Liston's bone forceps have a sharp point which could result in damage to the subcostal bundle or the pleura. For this reason, special rib shears have been designed. Vehmehren's rib holder and cutter is the most commonly used pattern. It consists of ring-shaped jaws, which are closed around the rib, and a blade which is separately driven through the rib by a separate handle. The Giertz rib holder is a similar instrument although it lacks a complete ring. It is hooked behind the rib and while outward traction is exerted the blade shears through the rib when the handles are closed.

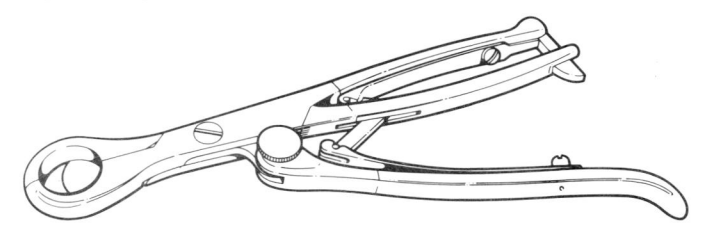

Fig.286 Vehmehren rib holder and costotome (Downs)

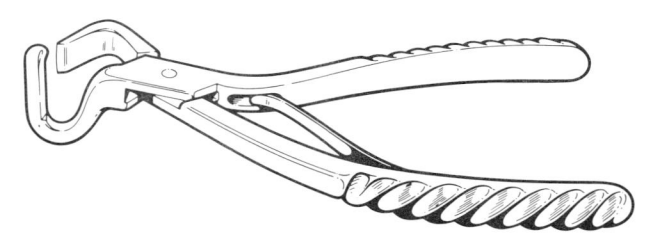

Fig.287 Doyen costotome (Downs)

13.10 Rib retractors and approximators

Rib and sternum retractors have to be very strong and there is no place for general surgical retractors. The choice is between the popular Finochietto, Tuffier, Blalock and Tudor-Edwards types. The Finochietto is probably the toughest and has interchangeable blades of various sizes.

Following thoracotomy it is necessary to approximate the ribs to relieve the strain on sutures. This is achieved by rib approximators. Roberts

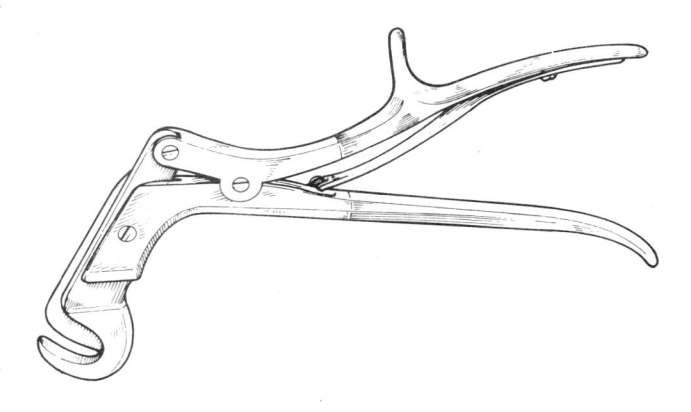

Fig.288 Giertz rib cutting shears (Downs)

VASCULAR AND THORACIC SURGERY   149

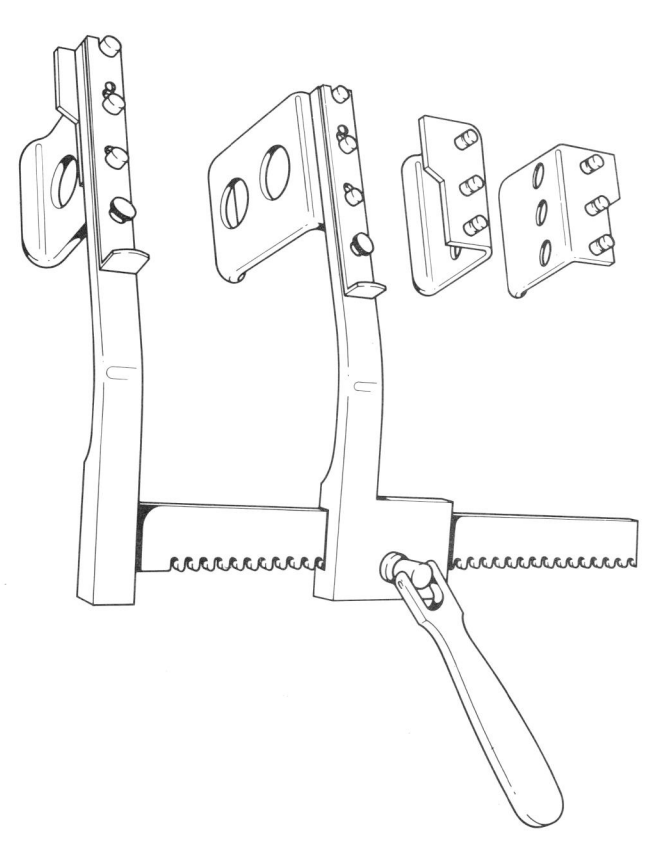

Fig.289 Burford Finochietto rib spreader (Downs)

Nelson's approximator was described in 1933 and consists of two levers joined by a bolt which can be quickly locked in position.

13.11 Oesophageal dilators

Prior to endoscopic stricture dilatation, oesophageal bougies were used both diagnostically and therapeutically. Dilators were often passed by patients

Fig.290 Price Thomas rib spreader (Downs)

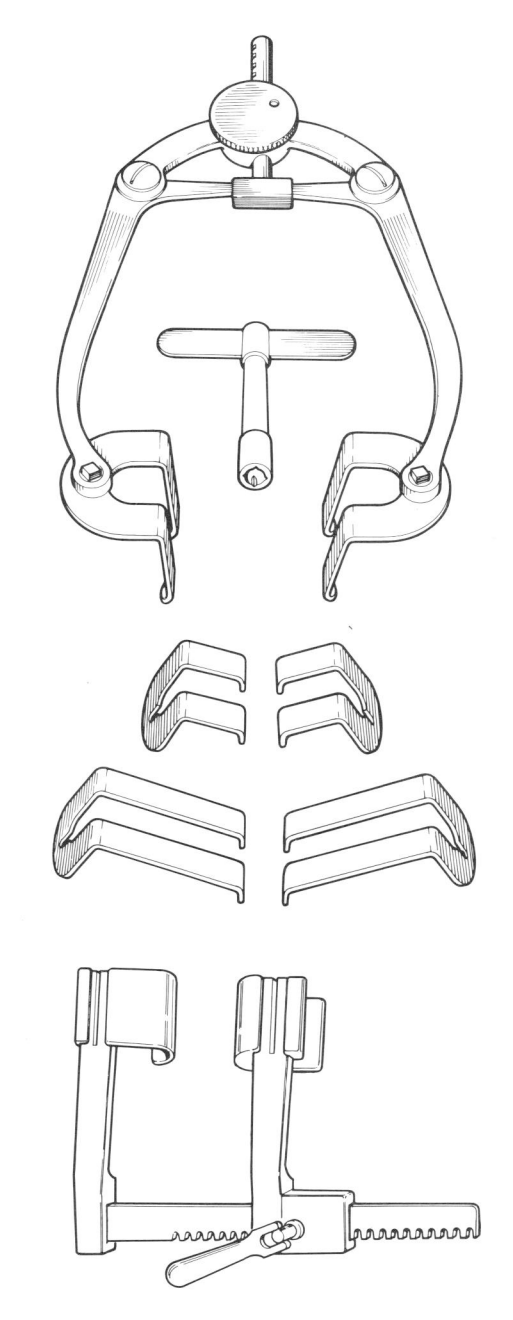

Fig.291 de Bakey rib spreader (Downs)

themselves. Early stricture dilators were made of gum elastic. The more recent of these are typified by Chevalier Jackson's dilators, used via a rigid oesophagoscope. Very narrow strictures were passed with a weighted silk thread which could then be used as a guide. These procedures were hazardous and difficult, and were carried out under general anaesthesia.

Before the introduction of Heller's operation, achalasia of the cardia was treated by a hydrostatic dilator, first introduced by Plummer. This comprised a rubber bag connected to a bougie. The bag was distended with water. The Negus bag was constructed on a similar principle.

Modern endoscopic stricture dilatation is carried out on sedated patients using the Eder–Puestow dilators. These were introduced before fibre-optic instruments. The dilatation set consists of a guide wire, the end of which has a flexible tip, and a set of graduated olive-shaped dilators, 21–54 French gauge. A new dilator has been introduced by Celestin which is made in one piece, is flexible and gradually increases in diameter from the tip proximally.

The procedure is carried out in left lateral position, as for diagnostic endoscopy. Under direct vision a guide wire is passed through the stricture. The endoscope is withdrawn leaving the guide wire *in situ*. The dilator is assembled, joining the leader to the bougie and flexible shaft, and these are threaded over the guide wire and pushed across the stricture. The dilator assembly is removed and a

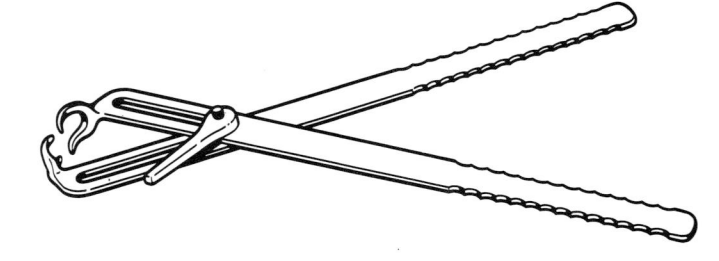

Fig.292 Roberts rib approximator (Downs)

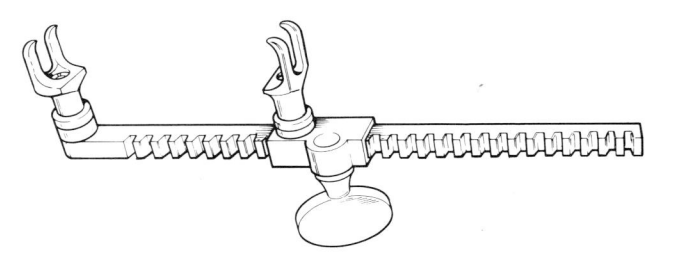

Fig.293 Sellors rib approximator (Downs)

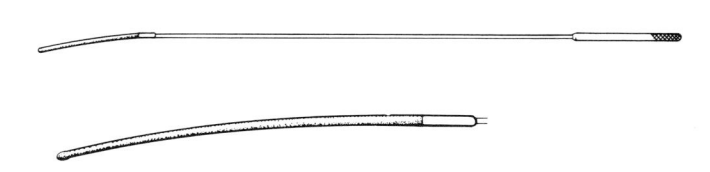

Fig.294 Jackson oesophageal bougie (Downs)

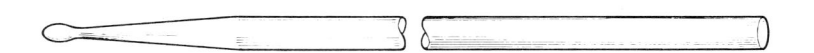

Fig.295 Neoplex oesophageal bougie (Downs)

larger olivary bougie passed, and so on until adequate dilatation has been achieved. The greatest danger of this procedure is perforation and this should be suspected if the patient complains of thoracic, cervical or upper abdominal pain.

Prestow, K.L. (1955) Conservative treatment of stenosing disease of the oesophagus. *Postgraduate Medicine*, **18**, 6.

Lilly, J.O. and McCaffery, T.D. (1971) Oesophageal stricture dilatation; a new method adapted to the fibreoptic oesophagoscope. *American Journal of Digestive Disease*, **16**, 1132.

Williamson, R.C.N. (1975) Peptic oesophageal stricture. *British Journal of Surgery*, **62**, 448-454.

Gear, M.W.L. (1981) Benign oesophageal strictures. In: *Therapeutic Endoscopy and Radiology of the Gut* (ed. Bennet, J.R.). Chapman and Hall, London.

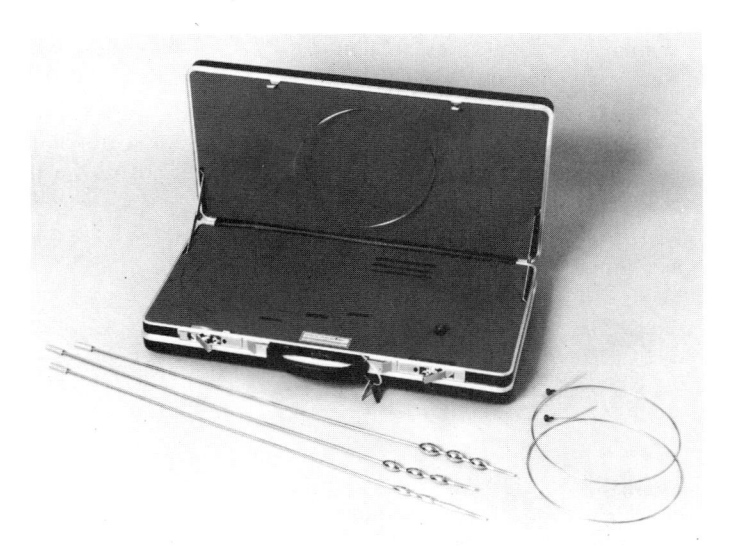

Fig.296 Key Med tri-dils triple olive oesophageal dilators set

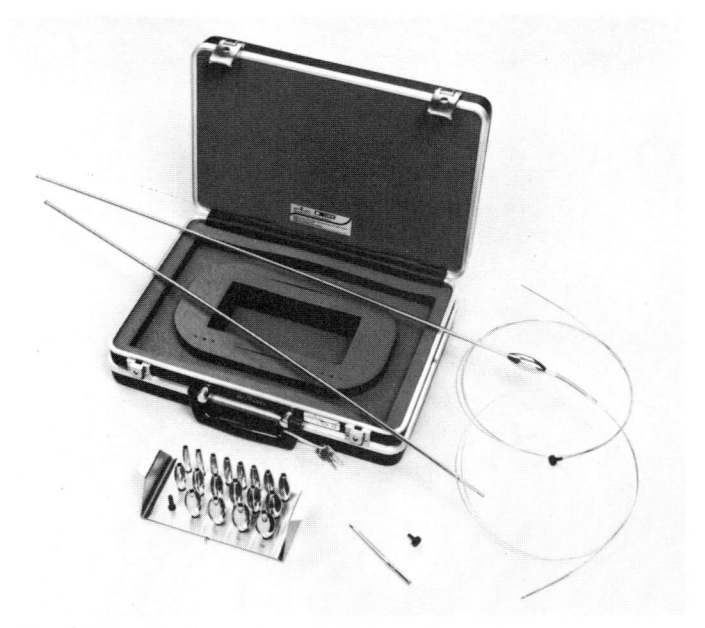

Fig.297 Key Med oesophageal dilators set

Chapter 14 Neurosurgery

14.1 Trephine and burr
14.2 Gigli saw
14.3 Bone rongeurs
14.4 Haemostats
14.5 Skull traction

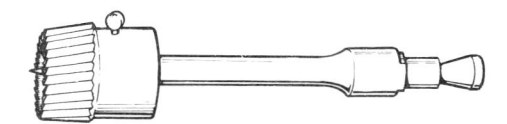

Fig.298 Rowbotham trephine (Downs)

14.1 Trephine and burr

The oldest neurosurgical operation is trephination of the skull. The trepan was an early predecessor of the trephine. It consisted of a crown saw for cutting small circular pieces of bone. The trephine, an improved version of the trepan, consists of a crown saw in the centre of which is an adjustable sharp steel pin which is fixed upon the bone to steady the operation. The saw is cone-shaped to prevent it from sudden plunging through when the full thickness of bone has been breached. Some trephines have adjustable guards to avoid this complication. The centre pin of the trephine, protruding approximately 2 mm, is pressed firmly against the bone and, by a twisting motion to and fro, a groove of sufficient size is made to keep the trephine steady. The central pin is then removed and sawing continued until the inner table of the skull is reached. The circular piece of bone can then be levered off. The instrument is driven by a handle, a brace (such as Hudson's) or a power drill. A simple opening may be made with a hand trephine, such as Horsley's. The trephine is used when a burr hole will not provide adequate

Fig.299 Buchanan trephine (Downs)

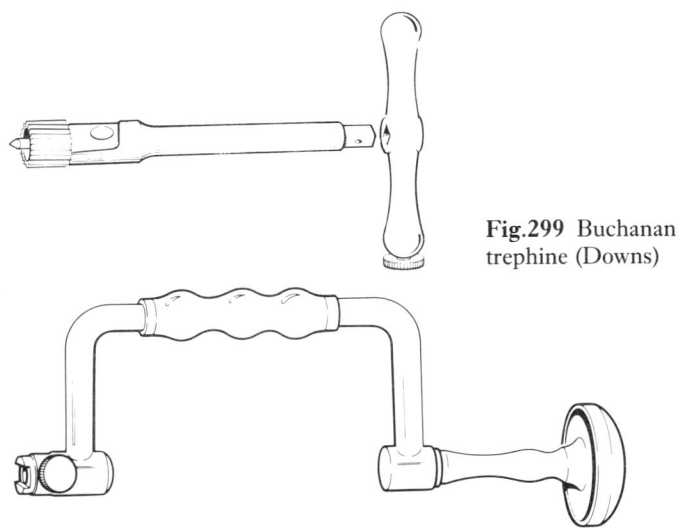

Fig.300 Hudson brace (Downs)

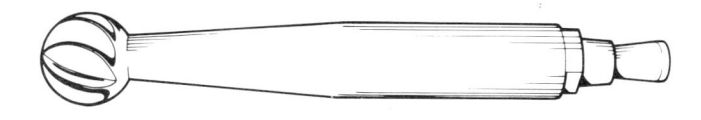

Fig.301 Hudson spherical burr (Downs)

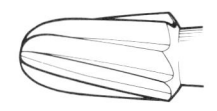

Fig.302 Hudson conical burr (Downs)

access and yet there is no need for craniotomy.

The alternative to the trephine is a burr. This is essentially a flat-ended drill which reduces the risk of injury to the underlying structures. A perforator needed to cut through the hard outer table of the skull before the burr is used. Burr holes are used for rapid decompression of the cranium or for the formation of formal craniotomy.

14.2 Gigli saw

Leonardo Gigli designed the wire saw in 1898 for symphisiotomy. It was a piece of iron wire with a double screw thread cut into it and detachable handles at each end. Later its potential was realised in neurosurgery for raising skull flaps. In its original design the saw had a tendency to break, and it was replaced by a plated and woven steel wire by Olivercrona.

The purpose of the saw is to enable the surgeon to cut the skull bone between two adjacent burr holes. The saw is passed between the dura and the inner table of the skull from one burr hole to the other. The de Martel's director was designed to facilitate this manoeuvre, as well as serving to protect the underlying dura during sawing. It is a curved flat steel director with blunt ends and a hook on its concave surface for the attachment of one end of the wire saw. The handles are T or ring shaped with hooks for the saw ends. The Gigli saw may also be used for sternal split.

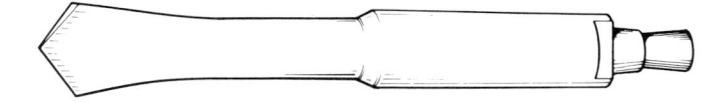

Fig.303 Hudson perforator (Downs)

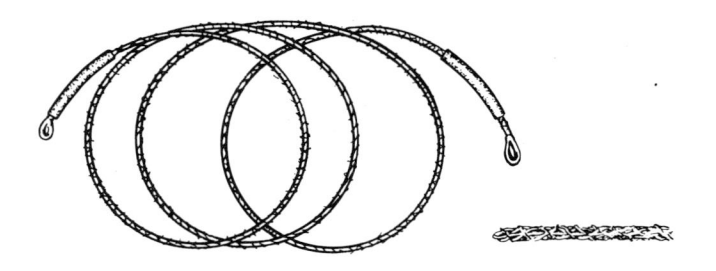

Fig.304 Gigli saw (Downs)

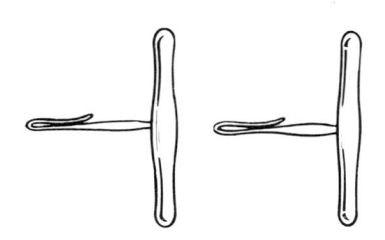

Fig.306 Gigli saw handles (Downs)

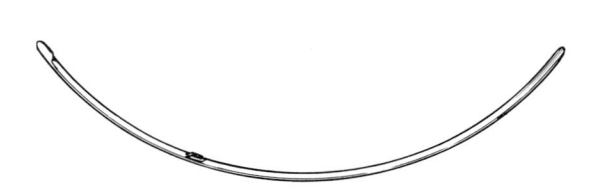

Fig.305 de Martel Gigli saw guide (Downs)

14.3 Bone rongeurs

For obvious reasons, there is little place for chisels and gouges in neurosurgical operations. Two trephine or burr holes can be connected by means of a saw, such as Gigli's. Hey's saw, although no longer in use, served the same purpose. William Hey described it in 1803. It resembles a two-bladed axe. One of the cutting edges is round and the other straight.

Enlargement of a single hole can be achieved using rongeurs, or nibbling forceps, although these can also be used for removing or shaping any bone. These are robust forceps with small jaws and long handles. The jaws are usually cup shaped. The top jaw is designed for cutting while the lower jaw is firmly held under the inner surface of the skull to prevent injury to the underlying structures. To reduce the force required to cut through the bone, some rongeurs have a double-action joint, similar to Payr's intestinal clamp. Rongeurs, such as Falconer's or Duggan's, resemble punch biopsy forceps. The right-angled jaws project from two parallel bars, one of which slides over the other when the handle is squeezed. These are suitable for finer work.

14.4 Haemostats

The scalp is very vascular and bleeds perfusely because the blood vessels lie in its connective tissue layer and when divided retract between the fibrous

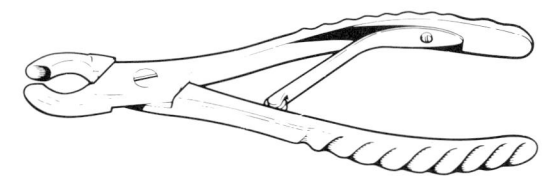

Fig.307 Horsley rongeur (Downs)

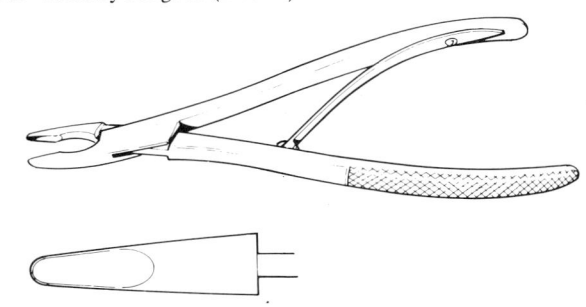

Fig.308 Cairns rongeur (Downs)

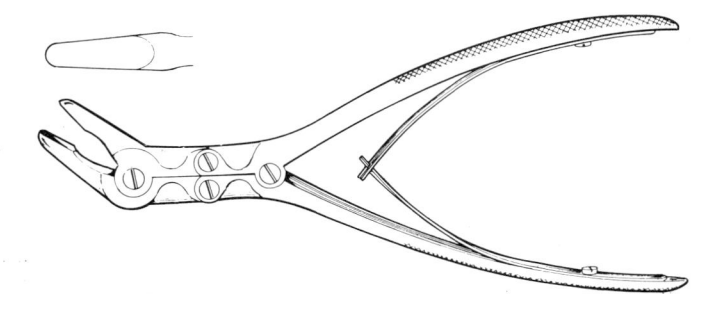

Fig.309 Killearn rongeurs (Downs)

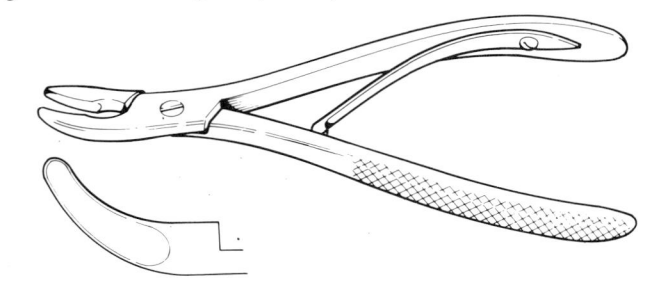

Fig.310 Pennybacker rongeur (Downs)

septa and do not contract in the usual manner.

One of the oldest techniques of controlling scalp bleeding is the application of a tourniquet. Godwin's tourniquet, also known as Chiene's, is a flexible metal band, one end of which is fixed to a metal block. The mobile end is adjusted by a pin and screw. It was placed round the head just above the ears to stem the branches of major scalp vessels. The same can be achieved with a simple rubber tourniquet.

Many different types of haemostatic forceps have been designed specifically for scalp haemostasis. Sargent's forceps, for example, have two transverse blades, one of which is placed beneath the scalp edge while the other compresses the skin margin from above. However, fine artery forceps, such as Cushing's, are perhaps better because they control bleeding points without any damage to the skin. Even less obtrusive are scalp clips made in different shapes and sizes and applied with clip forceps. Artery forceps, however fine, are unsuitable for the control of bleeding cerebral vessels. Cushing's silver clips and their modern successors are suitable for this purpose. They are V-shaped clips and are applied with clip-applying forceps.

14.5 Skull traction

Skull traction is indicated in spinal injuries for the reduction of fractures, dislocations and fracture-dislocations

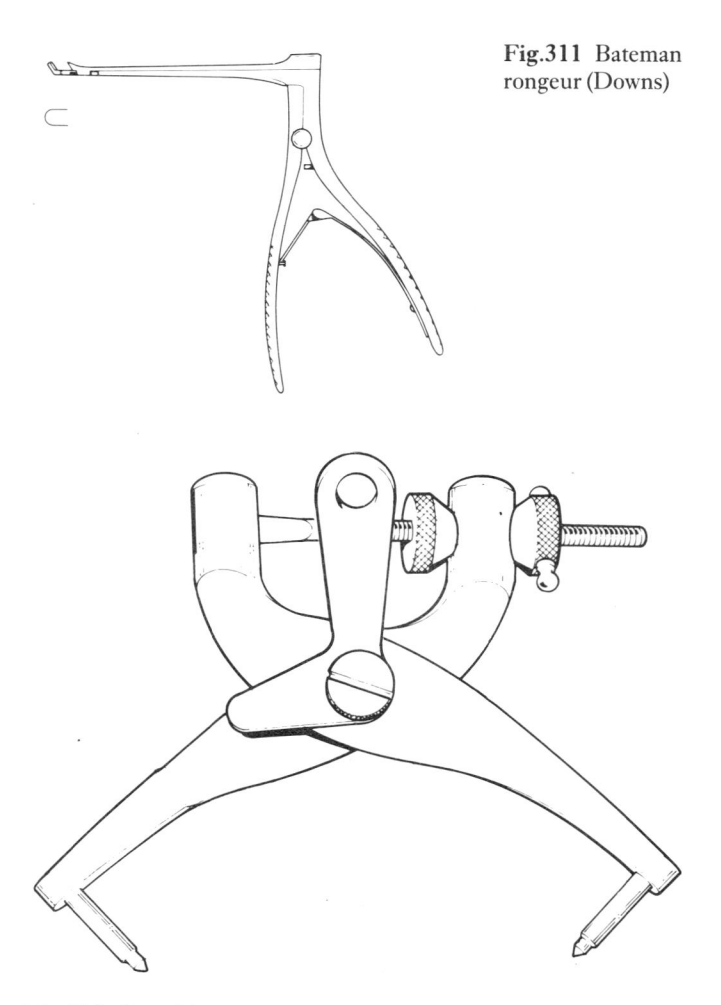

Fig.311 Bateman rongeur (Downs)

Fig.312 Crutchfield skull tongs (Downs)

of the cervical spine. It is also important for the maintenance of reduction and in the assistance of postural nursing of spinal injuries. The simplest skull tongs are those of Crutchfield. They are made in the form of robust forceps connected by a screw joint. The jaws are fitted with steel pins, at right angles to the jaws, pointing inward. The pins are shouldered, to limit their penetration. The opposite end of the instrument contains a screw between the two ends, fixed to one end. The approximation or retraction of the jaws is controlled by two nuts. Traction is applied to a metal piece which is fixed to the screw joint. Some Crutchfield tongs have modified steel pins whose angle, in relation to the jaws, can be altered by adjustment screws. The addition of a notch to steel pins has the advantage that their angle need not be adjusted as they hook into the outer table of the skull. The Blackburn skull caliper consists of two jaws which move along a transverse bar. Their distance from each other is adjustable and the angle of the pins is fixed. Traction is exerted via a hook which moves along the transverse bar.

The points on the skull are chosen, with the tongs maximally opened, on the coronal line, in front of the coronal line if extension is required, or behind the coronal line if flexion is needed. The points are clearly marked on the scalp and infiltrated with a local anaesthetic. A small incision is made with a scalpel blade over one of the marked points. The periosteum is elevated with a periosteal dissector. Using the Crutchfield guarded drill, a hole 3–4 mm deep is drilled in the outer table of the skull. The open caliper point is then inserted into the drilled hole and the position of the second incision is checked. The same procedure is carried out for the opposite side. The caliper is first inserted into one hold and then into the opposite hole. The tongs are tightened and secured with the counter nut.

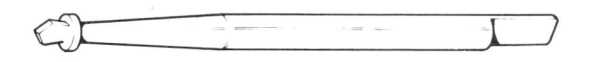

Fig.313 Crutchfield guarded perforator (Downs)

General Reading

Mitchell-Heggs, F. & Drew, H. G. R. (1963) *The Instruments of Surgery*. Heinemann, London.

Bennion, E. (1979) *Antique Medical Instruments*. Philip Wilson Publishers, London.

Farquhanson, E. L. (1939) *Illustrations of Surgical Treatment: Instruments and Applicances*. William & Wilkins, Baltimore.

Thompson, C. J. S. (1942) *History and Evolution of Surgical Instruments*. Schumann, New York.

Kirk, R. M. (1973) *Basic Surgical Techniques*. Churchill Livingstone, Edinburgh.

Index

Abdominal drains 53–4
Adam's saw 133
Adson's dissecting forceps 110
Allen–Brown shunt 47
Alms skin retractor 111
Amputation
  instruments 145–6
  knives 83
  saws 133
Anastomotic dehiscence 103
Aneurysm needles 144–5
Angioplasty, percutaneous
    transluminal 42–3
Arbuthnot Lane twin intestinal
    clamp 90
Argon laser 68
Argyle chest drain 54
Artery forceps 86
Arthrodax orthopaedic cast wire 139
Arthroscope 17–18
Asepsis 71
Autoclaving 71

Bakes bile duct dilators 100
Balfour retractor 97
Baycast 138
Bigelow evacuator 127
Biliary drains 60
Biopsy 27
  brush 28
  Crosby–Kugler intestinal 32
  high-speed drill 31
  needle 28–9
  punch forceps 29–30
  trephine 30–1
Bistouries 83–4
Blackburn skull caliper 157
Bladder
  evacuator 127
  stone sounds 117
Blair knife 111
Bone
  fixation 135–7
  instrument 133–5
  rongeurs 155
Bougies 117–18

Brodie's fistula probe-director 93
Bronchoscope 5–6
Bronchus clamps 146
Broviac catheter 40
Brush biopsy 28
Burr 153–4
Buselmeier shunt 47
Butcher saw 133

Cannulae, vascular 38–41
Cardiovascular instruments 142
Catgut 73
Catheter introducers 123
Catheter-over-guidewire 40
Catheter-over-needle 39
Catheters
  Broviac 40
  drum cartridge 39
  embolectomy 41–2
  Fogarty balloon 41
  Güntzig 42–3
  Hickman 41
  materials 56
  peritoneal dialysis 58–9
  pulmonary artery flotation 46–7
  tips 57
  urological 55–8
  vascular 38–41
Catheter-through-cannula 40
Catheter-through-needle 39
Caval filters 44–6
Celestin dilators 150
Cerclage 137
Cetrimide 72
Chest drains 54–5
Chisels, orthopaedic 134
Chlorhexidine 72
Chlorine 72
Cholangiography, percutaneous
    transhepatic 60
Cholecystectomy instruments 98–100
Choledochoscope 14–15
Clamps
  bronchus 146
  cardiovascular 142
  intestinal 89–92

Cleveland pedicle needle   145
Clips, scalp   156
Clutton's dilating sounds   117
CO_2 laser   68
Colonoscope   13–14
Computerised axial tomography   24–5
Cooper's hernia bistoury   84
Crosby–Kugler intestinal biopsy   32
Crutchfield skull tongs   156–7
Cryobiopsy   33
Cryosurgery   65–7
Curette   27
Cystometry   25
Cystostomy, percutaneous suprapubic   57
Cystourethrography   26
Cysto-urethroscope   18–19
Cytology   27

de Martel
   crushing clamp   92
   director   154
de Pezzer catheter   57
Deaver's retractor   95
Denham pin   137
Dennis Browne retractor   97
Dermatomes   111–12
Desjardins forceps   99
Dettol   72
Diathermy   63–4
   snare and loop   32
Directors   92–3
   de Martel   154
Disinfection   71–3
Dissecting forceps   89
Dissectors   92–3
Doppler effect ultrasound   22
Dormia stone extractor   128
Dornier extracorporeal shock wave lithotripsy   69–70
Doyen intestinal clamp   90
Drains
   abdominal   53–4
   biliary   60
   chest   54–5

Drum cartridge catheter   39
Drum dermatome   112

Eder–Puestow dilators   150
EEA stapling guns   104
Electrocautery   63
Ellik evacuator   127
Embolectomy catheters   41–2
Embolisation, therapeutic   43–4
Endarterectomy instruments   142–3
Endotracheal tubes   61–2
Ethylene oxide   72
Eve intestinal forceps   90

Fergusson's saw   133
Fibrescope   9
File   134
Filters
   caval   44–6
   Greenfield   45
Fluoroscopy   23
Fogarty balloon catheter   41
Foley balloon catheter   56
Forceps
   artery   156
   biopsy punch   29–30
   bone-cutting   135
   bone-holding   135
   cardiovascular   142
   dissecting   89
   Eve intestinal   90
   gall-bladder   99
   haemostatic   85–6, 156
   renal stone   124
   thumb   89
   tissue   110
   tissue-grasping   86–9
Formalin   72

Gall-bladder forceps   99
Garotte   37
Gas insufflator   16
Gastric tubes   49

INDEX

Gastroduodenoscope 8–10
Gastrointestinal endoscopy 7–14
GIA stapling instrument 106
Giertz rib holder 148
Gigli saw 154
Gillies needle holder 109
Gloves 75
Godwin's tourniquet 156
Goligher's sternal-lifting retractor 98
Gordon hook 111
Gouges 134
Greenfield filter 45
Güntzig catheter 42–3

Haemodialysis 47
Haemostatic forceps 85–6
Haemostats 155–6
Harris's needle and needle holder 125
Hexacholorphane 72
Hexcelite 138
Hey Groves bone-holding forceps 135
Hickman catheter 41
High-speed drill biopsy 31
Hip joint, artificial 79
Hoffman frame 136
Hopkins rod-lens telescope 18–19
Humby knife 111–12

Iglesias two-way irrigating
    resectoscope 120–1
Image intensifier 23–4
Implants 76–9
Intestinal clamps 89–92
Intestinal tubes 49
Intra-aortic balloon pump 48
Iodine 72
Ivalon sponge 77

Joll thyroid retractor 100

Kelly retractor 95
Kidney stones 69–70

Kilner needle holder 110
Kirschner wire 138
Knives 83–4
    skin grafts 111–12
Kocher dissector 100
Kocher intestinal clamp 90

Lahey forceps 99
Langenbeck retractor 94
Laparoscope 15–17
Laryngoscope 3–4
Laser 67–9
LDS stapling instrument 106
Le Veen shunt 59
Lightcast 138
Limb traction 137–8
Lister's dilating sounds 117
Lithotripsy 69–70
Lithotrite 121–2
Lloyd-Davies retractor 95

Macdonald–Stiles dissector 92
MacEwen hernia needle 145
Macintosh laryngoscope 3
Magill laryngoscope 3
Malecot catheter 57
Mallet 134
Maryfield introducer 123
Mayo scissors 84
McIndoe
    forceps 110
    scissops 85
Mediastinoscope 7
Medullary nails 136
Menghini needle 28
Metal implants 78
Metzenbaum's scissors 85
Michel clips 101
Microscopes, operating 114–15
Microsurgical instruments 113–14
Miller–Abbott tube 49
Millin retractor 125–6
Minnesota four-lumen tube 51
Morris retractor 95

Moynihan forceps   99
Myers' vein stripper   141

Nasogastric tubes   49
Naunton Morgan needle holder   94
Needle
  biopsy   28−9
  holders   93−4
    plastic surgery   109−10
    prostatectomy   125−6
Needles
  aneurysm   144−5
  pedicle   144−5
  prostatectomy   125−6
Negus
  laryngoscope   4
  tracheostomy tube   61
Nelson's scissors   85
Neodymium YAG laser   68
Nephroscope   20
Nylon   74

Oesophageal dilators   149−51
Oesophageal speculum   4
Oesophageal tubes   49−52
Oesophagoscope   7−8
Operating microscopes   114−15
Optical lithotrite   122
Optical urethrotomy   119
Osteotome   134
Otis urethrotome   118

Pasteurisation   71
Payr clamp   91
Pedicle needles   144−5
Penrose drain   53
Percutaneous transluminal
    angioplasty   42−3
Peritoneal dialysis catheters   58−9
Peritoneo-venous shunt   59−60
Pharyngoscope   3−4
Plaster   138−9
  instruments   138−9

shears   139
Plastic sponge implants   77
Plates   136
Polydioxane (PDS)   74
Polyethylene   77
Polyglycolic acid   73
Polypropylene   77
Polytetrafluoroethylene (PTFE)   78
Pressure flow study   26
Probes   92−3
Proctoscope   11−12
Prostatectomy instruments   125−6
Pulmonary artery flotation
    catheters   46−7
Pulse echo   21
Pyelolithotomy
  instruments   123−4
  percutaneous   128−31

Q switching   68
Quinton−Dillard−Scribner shunt   47

Rasp   134
Rehfuss's tube   49
Renal stone forceps   124
Resectoscope   120−1
Retractors   94−8
  prostatectomy   125−6
  pyelolithotomy   124
  rib   148
  skin   110−11
Reverdin's needle   94
Rib
  raspatories   147
  retractors and approximators   148−9
  shears   147
RNOH trephine   31
Rongeurs   155
Rougine   147
Ryle's gastroduodenal tube   49

Samway anchor tourniquet   37
Sargent's forceps   156

INDEX

Sauerbruch sternal splitter   147
Saws   133
   Gigli   154
Scalp clips   156
Scalpels   83–4
Scissors   84–5
   cardiovascular   142
Screws   136
Sengstaken oesophageal tube   51–2
Shears
   plaster   139
   rib   147
Shunt
   external arteriovenous   47–8
   peritoneo-venous   59–60
Silicones   77–8
Silk   74
Silverman needle   29
Skeletal traction   137–8
Skin
   retractors   110–11
Skin traction   137
Skull
   tongs   156–7
   traction   156–7
Sounds   117–18
Spark gap generator   63
Staff   117
Stainless steel suture   74
Stapling instruments   103–7
Starch powder   75
Steam   71
Steinmann pin   137
Sterilisation   71–3
Sternum-splitting instruments   146–7
Stones, basket extractors   128
Stryker oscillating saw   133
Suction drains   53
Sump drains   54
Surgical gloves   75
Sutures   73–4
   requirements for   76

TA stapling instrument   105
Teflon   77

Telescopes   16
   principles   18–19
Tetany   63
Thomas shunt   47
Thoracic instruments   146
Thumb forceps   89
Thyroid instruments   100–1
Tissue forceps   110
Tissue-grasping forceps   86–9
Tourniquet   37–8
   scalp bleeding   156
Tracheostomy tubes   61–2
Traction   137
   skull   156–7
Travers retractor   96
Trepan   30, 153
Trephine   153–4
   biopsy   30–1
Tru-cut biopsy needle   29
T-tubes   60
Tubes
   gastric and intestinal   49
   oesophageal   49–52
   tracheostomy and endotracheal   61–2
Turkel trephine   30
Tyndallisation   71

Ultrasound
   diagnostic   21–3
   pyelolithotomy   130
Underwater-seal bottle   55
Ureteroscope   20
Urethral pressure profile   25
Urethral sounds and bougies   117–18
Urethrotome   118–19
Urodynamics   25–6
Urological catheters   55–8
Urological endoscopy   18–20

Valve circuit generator   64
Vascular cannulae and catheters   38–41
Vascular prostheses   78
Vehmehren's rib holder and cutter   148
Vein strippers   141

Velour prosthesis   78
Venturi technique   5–6
Verres needle   16
Voiding cystourethrography   26
Volkmann's spoon   27

Watson Cheyne dissector   92
Wheelhouse staff   118
Wound
   healing   76
   retractors   94–8